5-Ingredient

STAGE 3 KIDNEY DISEASE DIET

Cookbook for Seniors

MARIANNE GREENE

ESSENTIALS EDITION

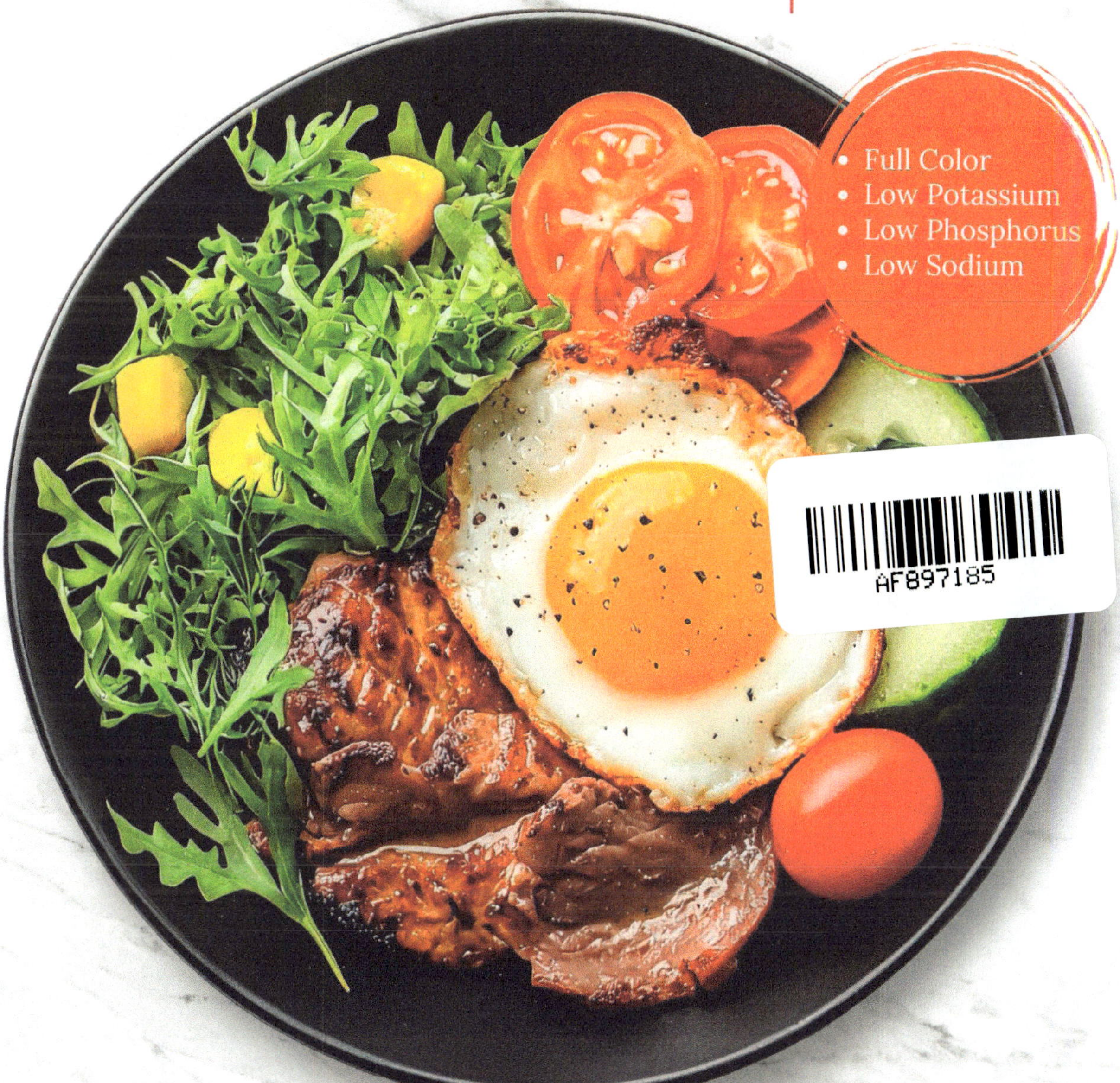

Disclaimer and Legal Notice

Important: This book is for informational purposes only and does not constitute medical, legal, or professional advice.

Neither the authors nor the publisher are medical professionals. The information in this book is not intended to replace medical advice, diagnosis, or treatment by a qualified healthcare provider. Always consult a qualified healthcare provider before starting or changing any treatment.

The publisher and authors disclaim all liability for any loss, injury, or damage incurred as a direct or indirect result of the use and application of any content in this book.

No warranty or guarantee, express or implied, is given regarding the accuracy, completeness, or suitability of the content. Laws and regulations change frequently; the reader is solely responsible for ensuring compliance with all applicable laws and for seeking professional advice as needed.

By using this book, you accept these terms and hold the publisher and authors harmless from any and all liability.

TABLE OF CONTENTS

TABLE OF CONTENTS

RECIPES

RECIPES

BONUS: Free Kidney-Safe Power Tools

Worried about dining out with Stage 3 Kidney Disease? We've got you covered. Grab your FREE Kidney-Safe Power Tools featuring:

- A game-changing Dining Out Cheat Sheet with smart swaps to order anywhere, red-flag items to avoid, and simple questions to ask your server.
- A CKD do-it-yourself Weekly Meal Planner to stay on track
- A Kidney-Friendly Grocery List for Smart Shopping
- Take control beyond your kitchen by starting with your bonus gift.

Click here to get your bonuses and our next book for FREE:

https://greenhopex.com/dining-out-s3kd

or Scan this QR code to Claim your free gifts:

Simple tools. Big impact. Better living starts in your pantry.

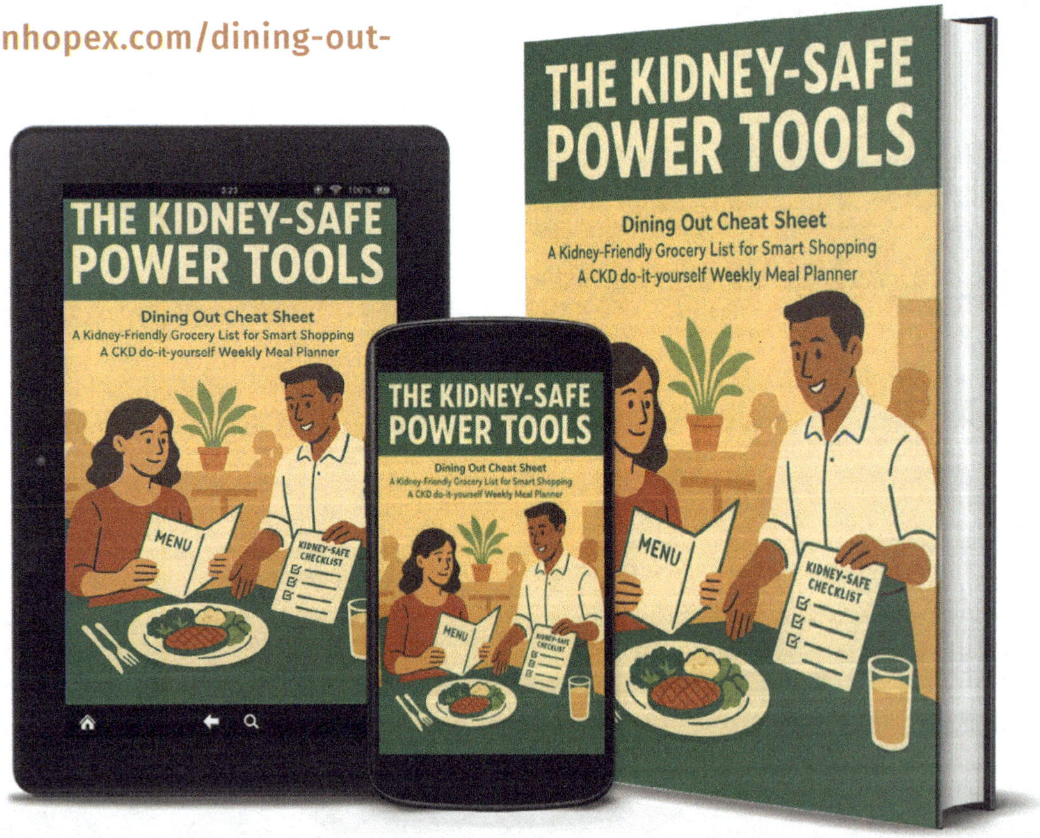

Join Our Private Facebook Group!

Living with CKD can feel isolating and overwhelming, especially when it comes to diet and lifestyle changes. In this group, you're not alone. You'll gain support from a community that truly understands what you're facing, get answers to your questions, and feel empowered with encouragement and resources tailored to your needs. Just search

"Kidney Disease Warriors: Stage 3 & 4 CKD Diet, Recipes and Community"

The group is on Facebook—we can't wait to welcome you.

Or Scan this and request to join our group <3

Authors Note

Dear Reader,

I want to begin with a warm welcome and a heartfelt thank you for picking up this book. Whether you found it in a hurry, on a difficult day, or while searching for hope and practical answers, I hope you'll feel at home here from the very first page. This book isn't just a collection of recipes or a list of do's and don'ts—it's an invitation to start fresh, feel empowered, and rediscover good food even in the face of stage 3 kidney disease.

Let me introduce myself. My name is Marianne Greene. For over seventeen years, I've worked as a senior caregiver in assisted living homes. I've spent days and nights supporting families, comforting folks through changes, and finding small ways to make life easier and more enjoyable. But nothing prepares you for when the diagnosis lands in your own family. That's what happened to me: My husband was told he had stage 3 chronic kidney disease. Suddenly, I wasn't just the helper—I was the wife, the partner, the cook, and the one with all the questions and worries.

I am not a nurse, nor am I a doctor. I am someone who has lived through the uncertainty and the everyday challenges of CKD, right alongside the people I love. I've cooked countless meals, swapped stories with other caregivers, and learned by living—one meal, one appointment, one new day at a time. When my husband was first diagnosed, I did what so many of you are probably doing now: I dove into books, scoured the internet, grilled the dietitians, and did everything I could to build up my knowledge and confidence. I wanted to know: How can I help him stay healthy—and happy? How can I make sure that our table is still a place for comfort and togetherness, not just restrictions and fear?

Out of that journey, this book was born.

Why This Book Exists

There are a lot of resources out there about chronic kidney disease, and a lot of them are overwhelming. Heavy textbooks, technical jargon, long lists of "never eat this" and "don't even think about that." Some cookbooks promise the world, but leave you feeling lost in the kitchen, or stuck with recipes that use rare ingredients and complicated steps. I know from experience that what most people need—especially at the start of their CKD journey—is something approachable. Something you can pick up today, flip through, and actually use to make your next meal.

This book is for the doers. For the family members and caregivers who want practical answers. For seniors who want to enjoy their food and keep their independence, without spending all day in the kitchen. For anyone who's ever looked at a complicated dietary plan and thought, "There has to be a simpler way."

If you're here, you're probably ready to get started, not get buried in details. That's why I've made every effort to keep things clear, simple, and encouraging.

What This Book Is (and Isn't)

I want to be upfront: This book is designed as a quick start guide—a friendly "on-ramp" for anyone feeling lost at the beginning of their stage 3 CKD journey. I wanted to provide some recipes and make this book affordable. I provide a good start for anyone to understand what they are dealing with and how to EVALUATE recipes and their diet.

BUT...

It isn't meant to be an exhaustive or deeply medical text.

Instead, you'll find what you need most right now: easy recipes, straightforward guidance, and a dose of reassurance.

If you're looking for MANY more tasty and 5 ingredient recipes, a detailed meal plan spanning months, please know this is just the beginning.

I am currently working on a more comprehensive recipe book with 100+ recipes and 60 day meal plans (and maybe, by the time you're reading this, it's already available—so feel free to search for my name, Marianne Greene, and see what's out there!).

UPDATE: It just got published, here it is: https://amzn.to/4lrPYoV

click this above to get your paperback of the book. Here is the QR code for the paperback of the main book in the series.

CKD just got so much easier at the price of a Starbucks coffee. <3

That upcoming book will offer extended meal plans, deeper explanations, and far more recipes for every taste and need. But I didn't want to wait until everything was "perfect" before helping people get started—so I put together this quick-start cookbook to get you moving in the right direction, fast.

What Makes my Books Different

You'll notice a few things about the recipes and advice in these pages:

- All Ingredients are Grocery Store Staples: I know what it's like to scan a recipe and wonder, "Where on earth do I buy that?" Every ingredient in this book is something you'll find at a regular grocery store—no specialty shops, no chasing down rare or expensive items.
- Max 5 Main Ingredients Per Recipe: Because simplicity is sanity. Most of us don't have the energy (or the patience) for complicated dishes. Every recipe here is built around five main ingredients or fewer, with maybe a handful of pantry items you already have on hand.
- Easy to Chew: Many seniors, and people with CKD, have trouble chewing or swallowing. Every recipe was tested with this in mind. I've

focused on tender textures, gentle flavors, and meals that are truly pleasant and easy to eat.

- **All Recipes Under 30 Minutes:** You won't find slow-cooked stews that take hours or intricate baking projects. Every meal in this book can be made from start to finish in under half an hour. Because when you're hungry, or tired, you need something now—not later.
- **Low-Effort Prep, Minimal Equipment:** No fancy tools, no confusing steps. If you can use a knife, a pan, and an oven—or even just an air fryer—you can cook every meal in this book.

How to Use This Book

If you're feeling overwhelmed, I want you to know: you don't have to read this cover to cover in one sitting. Start wherever you are—maybe you want to flip straight to the recipes, or maybe you want to read through the quick tips and background information. However you use this book is the right way.

Take what you need, skip what doesn't fit, and don't be afraid to make adjustments for your own comfort and needs. Every recipe is adaptable—try different herbs, adjust textures, swap proteins, and make it your own. The goal isn't perfection, it's progress and pleasure.

I also encourage you to share this book—with your family, your friends, your healthcare team. If you have a dietitian or doctor helping you, show them the recipes and nutrition counts. This book is meant to be a resource, a jumping-off point, and a conversation starter. The more support you have, the easier this journey will feel.

A Personal Message—From My Table to Yours

I wish I could sit down across from you, share a cup of tea, and hear your story. I know what it's like to feel lost and worried, and I know the comfort that a good meal, shared with people you love, can bring.

When my husband was diagnosed, I felt like the ground had shifted beneath us. Despite all my years working in senior care, I was scared. I wanted answers, but mostly, I wanted to feel in control again—to give him something nourishing and delicious that would support his health, not just fill his stomach. That's why I wrote this book. Every recipe here is something that made a difference in our life—something that brought a little normalcy, a little pleasure, and a lot of hope to our days.

Over time, I've seen how even small changes—simpler meals, more thoughtful shopping, keeping track of key nutrients—can lead to better lab numbers, more energy, and brighter moods. I've cooked for friends, neighbors, and residents in

A NOTE ABOUT PROGRESS AND PERFECTION

You might be feeling pressure to "get it right," to follow every rule, to never slip up. I want to let you off the hook—no one is perfect, and no plan should make you miserable. This book is here to help you start, not to police every bite or add guilt to your plate. Celebrate every win, no matter how small. Even just reading this, you're already taking a powerful step for your health.

assisted living homes, and I've watched the same thing happen: When food feels manageable, life feels a little less daunting.

Looking Ahead—A Full Guide Is Coming Soon

In my upcoming book, you'll find practical tools and support to help you manage your kidney health with confidence. Sign up to download a free gift from the book and be notified when it's released.

Here's what to expect:

- 60-Day Meal Plan: A complete plan to take the guesswork out of your meals—follow it as is or mix and match.
- 80+ Easy, Delicious Recipes: Designed with overlapping ingredients to simplify shopping and reduce waste.
- Detailed Nutritional Info: Every meal includes key facts like calories, protein, potassium, phosphorus, sodium, fat, carbs, cholesterol, and oxalates—plus daily totals.
- Expanded Guidance: Includes deeper nutritional advice, full shopping lists, and support for caregivers and families.
- Culturally Diverse Options: Recipes for different dietary needs and preferences.

This book is just the beginning—I'd be honored to support you on your journey. Reach out anytime to share your story or ask questions.

Love and Gratitude

Above all, I want you to know that you're not alone. Whatever brought you to this book—concern for yourself, for a loved one, for your patients or friends—you're part of a community of people who care, learn, and adapt together. You can find the link to our facebook group and the QR code in the "Resources" chapter. Or just search "Kidney Disease Warriors: Stage 3 & 4 CKD Diet, Recipes and Community" on Facebook—we can't wait to welcome you.

I hope to see you there. And hopefully you will find comfort, clarity, and even joy in these pages.

Thank you for letting me join you, even in a small way, on your path toward better health and good food. From my kitchen to yours—wishing you easy meals, happy days, and steady progress.

With all my love,

Marianne Greene <3

P.S.

If the pictures look great, it's because they were made in a kitchen studio, perfect lighting and high tech cameras, don't get discouraged if yours don't look like them. They'll be just as tasty.

If you enjoy these recipes, if you find the meal plans helpful, or if you want to share your own ideas, I would love to hear from you. You can find updates, resources, and news about my upcoming books by searching my name online. Together, we can make CKD management a little more welcoming, a little less lonely, and a lot more delicious.

The Senior's Essential Guide to Stage 3 CKD

Step 1: Welcoming Change with Knowledge and Hope

Imagine sitting by a window with your favorite cup of tea. The sunlight feels warm, but a letter from your doctor sits on the table: "You have stage 3 chronic kidney disease." Maybe you expected this, or maybe it caught you off guard. Either way, you feel a flurry of questions—What now? What does this mean for my daily life?

Let's pause for a moment. Take a deep breath. This is a new chapter, not the end of your story.

Millions of people live with CKD, and many thrive by making small, steady changes. You have more power than you might think. This book isn't about overwhelming you with new information—it's about clarity and control, about feeling better, and keeping the things you love: time with family, good meals, independence, and hope.

Throughout these chapters, you'll find stories, tips, and gentle guidance. There's no rush; go at your own pace. Take each step as it comes. The journey is yours, and you have support every step of the way.

Step 2: Meet Your Kidneys—The Unsung Heroes

Let's get acquainted with your kidneys. They're about the size of a fist, nestled deep in your lower back. These organs don't get the fanfare of your heart or brain, but they're quietly essential. Imagine them as two hard-working housekeepers, sifting and sorting your blood, removing waste, balancing fluids, and keeping things just so.

Now, as we age, it's common for kidneys to slow down a bit—just like everything else. But CKD, or chronic kidney disease, means the filtering job is getting tougher for them, and sometimes, waste and extra fluid can start to build up.

There are five stages of CKD. If you're reading this, you or someone you care about is likely in stage 3—a middle ground. Your kidneys are working at about 30–59% of their normal capacity. It's not ideal, but it's also not hopeless. This is the stage where awareness and action can make a world of difference.

A doctor determines your CKD stage using something called GFR, or glomerular filtration rate. Think of GFR like a kitchen sieve: a new one lets water run through easily, but as it gets clogged, water moves more slowly. A lower GFR means more "clogging." But it's not too late to keep things moving!

Stage 3 breaks down even further:

- Stage 3a: Your GFR is between 45 and 59.
- Stage 3b: It's between 30 and 44.

This nuance helps your care team tailor advice, but what matters most for you is knowing that every good choice you make can help slow the loss of function and help you keep living well.

Step 3: Listening to Your Body—Symptoms, Signals, and Progress

Here's a comforting truth: many people with early CKD feel completely normal. That's because kidney disease is often called a "silent" condition. The signs can be so subtle—fatigue that's easy to blame on age, swelling that sneaks up on you, a little more itching, maybe some changes in urination. Sometimes there's a loss of appetite, a little nausea, or foggy thinking.

Picture a houseplant that's slowly not getting enough water. It doesn't wilt overnight; it changes slowly, day by day. CKD can be just as gentle, almost invisible at first.

But awareness is your best tool. When you know what to look for, you can act early. Let's gently review some possible symptoms:

- Swelling in your ankles, feet, or hands—like putting on shoes and noticing they're a bit tight.
- Feeling more tired, even when you're getting enough sleep.
- Going to the bathroom more, or less, than usual—or noticing foam or darker color in your urine.
- Itchy or dry skin that lotions don't quite solve.
- Feeling slightly short of breath, especially when moving around.
- Occasional dizziness or trouble focusing.

It's easy to shrug these off, but mentioning them to your doctor helps keep you on track.

Remember, CKD often travels with friends: high blood pressure, diabetes, or heart disease. They can speed up kidney damage if left unchecked, but with careful management, you can protect your kidneys and your overall health.

TThink about your recent days. Have you noticed anything new or different? Jot it down or share it with someone you trust. Every little note helps you and your care team put the puzzle together.

Step 4: Your Nutrition Compass—Turning Food into Medicine

Now, let's wander into your kitchen. What you eat is one of the most powerful ways you can support your kidneys—every meal, every snack, every choice, big or small.

A lot of advice out there sounds strict, maybe even joyless: "Don't eat this. Never touch that." But this isn't about giving up everything you love. It's about shifting, swapping, and discovering new favorites—about enjoying food that loves your kidneys back.

Let's start by understanding the "big four" nutrients your kidneys notice the most:

Protein, Sodium, Potassium, and Phosphorus.

Protein—Not Too Much, Not Too Little

Your muscles need protein for strength and healing, especially as you age. But when kidneys are struggling, excess protein creates more waste, making their job harder.

A simple rule: For people with Stage 3 CKD, getting the right amount of protein is key—not too high, not too low. A good daily target is about 0.3 to 0.4 grams of protein per pound of body weight (or 0.6 to 0.8 grams per kilogram).

For example, a senior woman weighing 180 pounds (about 82 kg) should aim for roughly 55 to 65 grams of protein per day.

Focus on variety:

- Lean chicken or turkey, eggs, fresh fish
- Tofu, beans, or unsalted nuts (in modest portions)
- Use a kitchen scale if you have one; otherwise, remember that a serving of meat is about the size of your palm.

Sodium—The Silent Saboteur

Sodium hides in more places than you'd expect—canned soups, breads, sauces, even breakfast cereal. Too much sodium raises blood pressure and causes fluid to build up, making your kidneys and heart work harder.

Aim for under 2,000 milligrams a day. Use herbs, garlic, lemon, or vinegar for flavor. Check labels: anything labeled "low sodium" (less than 140 mg per serving) is a better bet. Put down the salt shaker—you won't miss it for long.

Potassium—Balance is Key

Potassium helps your muscles and nerves function, but when kidneys falter, too much can become dangerous. Not everyone with stage 3 CKD needs to avoid potassium, but some do.

- If your doctor gives you a target (often 2,000 mg a day), keep these guidelines in mind:

- Enjoy apples, berries, grapes, and lettuce
-
- Use caution with bananas, oranges, potatoes, tomatoes
- Scan packaged foods for "potassium chloride"—if you see it, put it back on the shelf.

Phosphorus—The Hidden Mineral

Phosphorus is important for bones, but too much builds up when kidneys slow down. High phosphorus can make bones weak and itchy skin worse.

Phosphorus is especially sneaky in processed foods and dark sodas. Look for "phos" in ingredient lists: phosphoric acid, sodium phosphate, and so on. Aim for under 1,000 mg per day, and rely on fresh foods over packaged ones. As with potassium, some people need to limit phosphorus more than others.

Fluids—Finding the Right Balance

Most people with stage 3 CKD don't need to limit fluids unless told by their doctor. But pay attention to thirst, swelling, and urine output. Sip water throughout the day, and steer clear of sugary sodas or drinks with artificial sweeteners.

Calories—Fuel for Healing

You need enough calories to keep your energy up, maintain muscle, and avoid unwanted weight loss. Most adults need 30–35 calories per kilogram of body weight each day. If your appetite drops, try smaller, more frequent meals.

Pause and reflect: What is your favorite comfort food? How might you adapt it with these guidelines? What new ingredient would you like to try?

Step 5: The CKD-Friendly Kitchen—From Shopping List to Table

Imagine opening your pantry and seeing shelves stocked with safe, tasty, and easy-to-prepare foods. The CKD kitchen doesn't have to be restrictive. In fact, it can be an opportunity to rediscover flavors, textures, and meals that make you feel good—physically and emotionally.

Foods to Fill Your Plate

Focus on foods that love your kidneys:

- Grains: White rice, pasta, white or wheat bread, unsalted crackers, tortillas.
- Proteins: Skinless poultry, eggs, tofu, fresh fish, a few unsalted nuts.
- Dairy & Substitutes: Plain milk, unsweetened soy or rice milk, Greek yogurt, low-sodium cheese.
- Vegetables: Carrots, green beans, cucumbers, lettuce, bell peppers, cabbage, cauliflower.
- Fruits: Apples, berries, grapes, peaches, pears (fresh or canned in water).
- Healthy Fats: Olive oil, avocado, flaxseed oil, grass-fed butter or

ghee.

Keep your pantry ready with these basics:

- Olive oil, extra virgin and regular
- Vinegars: apple cider, white, red wine
- Lemon or lime juice (fresh or bottled)
- Garlic powder, onion powder, and dried herbs (basil, oregano, parsley, thyme, dill, rosemary)
- Spices like cinnamon, cumin, nutmeg, and paprika
- Baking powder, baking soda
- Honey, maple syrup (in moderation)
- Canned tomatoes (no salt added)

Foods to Limit

Some foods are best enjoyed rarely:

- Processed meats (hot dogs, bacon, sausages, deli meat)
- Canned foods with added salt
- Cheese spreads, American cheese, cottage cheese
- Salty snacks (chips, crackers, trail mixes)
- Sauces, condiments, and dressings high in sodium, phosphorus, or potassium
- Sodas, especially dark colas (phosphorus content)
- Foods with "phos-" or "potassium-" in the ingredients

Smart Swaps

A little creativity goes a long way:

- Try avocado or homemade hummus in place of cheese spreads.
- Use wild-caught fish or pasture-raised meats rather than processed ones.
- Unsweetened soy milk or rice milk can replace cow's milk.
- Sourdough bread is easier to digest and often lower in potassium than commercial whole grain bread.
- Swap out seasoned salt for blends of dried herbs and lemon zest.

Kitchen Tips for Seniors

Cooking should never feel like a chore.

- Use pre-chopped or frozen vegetables to save time and energy.
- One-pot meals and slow cookers reduce cleanup and let flavors mingle.
- Tools like jar openers, electric can openers, and grip pads can ease arthritis and make meal prep more enjoyable.
- If your energy is low, cook in short bursts, or make larger batches to freeze for later.

Pause and consider: What meals bring you comfort? How can you adapt them with these swaps or tips?

Step 6: Simple Routines for Lasting Kidney Health

Kidney health is built not just at the dinner table, but through daily rhythms—how you eat, how you move, how you rest, and how you manage the little stresses of life.

Portion Wisdom

"Eat the rainbow" is great advice, but so is "keep it simple."

The Balanced Plate Method is your friend:

Half your plate: low-potassium veggies

A quarter: lean protein (about the size of a deck of cards)

A quarter: kidney-friendly carbs (white rice, pasta, tortillas)

Let your plate guide you. No need for measuring cups at every meal—just a little visual awareness.

Meal Timing

Aim for regular, steady meals. Don't skip breakfast, and try to eat every 3–4 hours. This keeps energy steady and prevents overeating.

Small snacks—an apple, a boiled egg, a few unsalted crackers—can prevent blood sugar swings and keep you feeling satisfied.

Label Reading Made Easy

The world of packaged foods can be overwhelming, but a few simple rules help:

Look for sodium under 140 mg per serving.

Scan for "phos-" or "potassium-" in the ingredients.

The fewer the ingredients, the better.

Remember, the fresher the food, the fewer surprises.

Cooking for One or Two

If you live alone, cooking can feel like too much work. Try batch-cooking and freezing portions, or invite a friend or family member to share a meal prep day. One-pot meals, slow cooker recipes, and simple salads make it easy.

Staying Active

Gentle movement supports your kidneys and your energy:

Walk for 10–15 minutes daily—indoors or out

Try chair stretches or light yoga

Gardening, dancing, even tidying up counts

If you have arthritis or limited mobility, check with your doctor for safe exercises.

Pause: How do you feel after a walk, stretch, or moment of movement? Notice your energy and mood.

Step 7: Joyful Living—Eating Out, Socializing, and Celebrations

Life with CKD isn't just about rules—it's

about living fully, enjoying friends, and savoring moments big and small.

Eating Out

With a little planning, dining out is possible—and even fun:

- Call ahead and ask if dishes can be made with less salt or sauce on the side.
- Choose grilled, baked, or steamed options over fried or breaded.
- Ask for half portions, or share a meal with a friend.
- Bring your own kidney-friendly dish to potlucks or family gatherings.

Don't be shy—most restaurants want to help. And remember, what you eat most of the time matters more than any single meal.

Social Gatherings

Food is a way we connect. Don't let dietary changes keep you from participating.

- Eat a small, safe snack before events to avoid overindulging.
- Focus on the company, laughter, and conversation.
- Offer to bring a dish you know is CKD-friendly.

Your loved ones want you there. The joy of connection often outweighs the worry over food.

Mindful Indulgence

Every now and then, you might want a treat outside your plan. Enjoy it mindfully, savor each bite, and return to your routine at the next meal. One indulgence won't undo your progress.

Pause and reflect: What does joyful living look like for you? Is it a game night, a sunny walk, a family dinner? Picture yourself enjoying it fully.

Step 8: Building a Support Network

You don't walk this path alone. Think of your healthcare team as fellow travelers, ready to guide and encourage you.

Your Medical Team

- Primary care doctor: Keeps an eye on your whole health picture.
- Nephrologist: The kidney expert, guiding medication, lab tests, and treatment.
- Dietitian: Helps personalize your nutrition plan—don't hesitate to ask for a referral!

Bring questions to every appointment:

- Is my protein intake just right?
- Should I watch my potassium or phosphorus more closely?
- How often should we check my labs?
- Are my medications kidney-safe?
- Can we adjust my plan for more energy or comfort?

Keeping a Health Journal

Write down what you eat, drink, and how you feel—no need for perfection. Even a few notes about meals, fluids, and symptoms like swelling or fatigue provide clues.

This helps your doctors spot trends, troubleshoot issues, and celebrate your successes. It's like a personal map guiding your care.

Regular Check-Ins

Expect regular labs to check your GFR, creatinine, potassium, phosphorus, and urine protein. These guide your plan, but so does your voice: tell your team how you're feeling, what's working, and what you'd like to change.

Pause: Is there a question you've wanted to ask but haven't? Write it down and bring it to your next visit.

Step 9: Staying Motivated and Daily Joy

CKD is part of your story, not the whole of it. Small victories add up. Every healthy meal, every gentle walk, every good question brings you closer to your best possible health.

Mindset Matters

Focus on what you can do—not what you can't. Celebrate progress, not perfection. Maybe you drank a little more water today, took a walk, or tried a new recipe. That's a win.

Hydration—Just Right

Unless your doctor says otherwise, 6–8 cups of water daily is ideal. Use a glass bottle, sip slowly, and avoid relying only on thirst. Older adults often feel less thirsty, but steady hydration is vital.

Gentle Movement

Any movement counts:

A stroll outside, a dance in the kitchen, or gentle stretches by the TV

- If you're chair-bound, try seated exercises or leg lifts
- Movement isn't about sweat—it's about joy, flexibility, and strength.

Stress and Sleep

Stress can creep in, raising blood pressure and disrupting sleep. Take time each day to unwind:

- Try slow, deep breathing. Inhale for four, hold for four, exhale for four.
- Read, knit, listen to music, or look out the window with a cup of tea.
- Before bed, dim the lights, avoid screens, and let your mind settle.

Sleep is when your body repairs. Protect it as you would any precious medicine.

Pause and reflect: What is one small thing you can do today to care for your mind or body? Give yourself credit for every step.

Step 10: Holistic Health with CKD

When it comes to living well with kidney disease, food is just part of the picture. As we get older—especially with CKD in the mix—our bodies handle medications and supplements differently, making what's in our medicine cabinet just as important as what's in our fridge.

1. Medicines and CKD: A Delicate Balancing Act

Think of your kidneys as a filter that's gotten a bit slower with age. Many common medicines, including painkillers and blood pressure tablets, can build up in the body, sometimes causing more trouble than the problem they were meant to fix. It's not just prescription meds—everyday remedies like ibuprofen, certain antibiotics, or even that cheerful bottle of "herbal detox" can be risky.

Real-World Tips:

- Always bring an up-to-date medication list (including vitamins and over-the-counter pills) to every appointment. Keep a copy near the phone or in your wallet.
- Never stop or change a medicine because of something you saw on TV or a neighbor's advice—your doctor or pharmacist is your best source for what's safe for kidneys.

2. The "Natural" Trap: Not Everything Herbal Is Harmless

It's tempting to reach for supplements or herbal teas that promise to "boost your kidneys." Sadly, natural doesn't always mean safe. Even common antacids, cold meds, and laxatives can cause trouble for people with CKD. And some herbal blends can be downright dangerous (looking at you, "kidney cleanses" and anything with St. John's Wort).

Pro Tip:

Before starting any new supplement, vitamin, or over-the-counter product, ask your doctor or pharmacist for the kidney-safe seal of approval.

3. Supplements: Less Is Usually More

Older adults with CKD often see ads for miracle cures, bone boosters, or "energy in a bottle." Most of the time, your kidneys—and your wallet—are better off with only the essentials your doctor recommends. For example:

- Multivitamins should be kidney-friendly (low in potassium and phosphorus)
- Vitamin D, iron, or calcium—only if prescribed and in the right amount

Be cautious with high doses of vitamin C (can cause kidney stones)

Remember:

If it's not on your doctor's list, think twice. "More" doesn't mean "better"—especially for kidneys!

4. Making Medication

Management Simple (Even on Forgetful Days)

If you find yourself squinting at tiny pill labels, you're not alone. Try a weekly pill organizer, set phone alarms for reminders, or ask your pharmacy about easy-open bottles and blister packs. Share your system with a friend or family member—sometimes a friendly check-in is the best safety net.

5. Watch for Interactions—It's a Team Effort

The more pills or supplements, the higher the chance of drug interactions. Stick to one pharmacy if you can—they can help spot potential mix-ups. And always tell every doctor, nurse, or dentist your full medication list (yes, even the herbal tea bags!).

Warning Signs:

New nausea, confusion, skin rashes, or irregular heartbeats should never be ignored—call your doctor right away.

6. Regular Medication Reviews: Don't Wait for New Year's

Bring all your medicines—prescription, over-the-counter, and "natural"—to a review with your doctor or pharmacist at least twice a year. Ask if every pill is still needed and safe for your current kidney health.

7. Non-Drug Relief for Everyday Aches

Many common CKD symptoms (like pain, cramps, or trouble sleeping) can be managed with simple non-drug approaches:

- Heat packs or gentle stretching for pain
- Evening routines or soothing music for sleep
- Fiber-rich veggies and movement for constipation

8. Oral Health, Immunity, and Full-Body Wellness

Good oral health helps prevent infection and inflammation—so keep up with brushing, flossing, and regular dentist visits (let them know about your CKD).

Vaccines are your shield—don't skip flu, pneumonia, or COVID-19 shots. And if you get a cut or fever, act quickly and call your doctor.

9. Coordinating Care for Multiple Health Issues

If you're juggling CKD along with diabetes, heart issues, or arthritis, let all your doctors know about every medicine and lab result. A central folder or notebook helps keep instructions straight.

10. Staying Safe at Home (Because Gravity Is Not Our Friend)

Falls are more common as we age—and some CKD medicines can add to the risk. Keep walkways clear, use grab bars in the bathroom, and wear sturdy shoes with non-slip soles (even on "quick trips" around the house).

Fun Fact:

Decluttering the floor can reduce fall risk by up to 30%!

11. When to Reach Out—Never Hesitate

If you experience sudden swelling, confusion, chest pain, fever, or trouble peeing, call your doctor right away. Keep emergency numbers handy, along with your medication list.

12. You're Not Alone—Let Others Help

Share your care plan and medication list with someone you trust. Set up regular check-ins, even if it's just a friendly phone call. CKD support groups (many meet online or by phone) can be a lifeline for tips and encouragement.

Wrapping Up: Your Medication Know-How Is a Superpower

Managing medications and supplements safely is just as crucial as what's on your plate. Stay organized, ask questions, and partner with your healthcare team. Each small step you take is a big investment in your independence and peace of mind.

Step 11: Mental, Social, and Emotional Wellness with CKD

A CKD diagnosis brings changes, not just to your kidneys, but to your whole life—body, mind, and social circles included. For seniors, it can mean new routines, smaller social circles, or worries about independence. Here's how to make sure your heart, mind, and sense of humor stay just as strong as your health plan.

1. Emotions: All Aboard the Rollercoaster

Fear, sadness, anger, denial, and even relief—whatever you're feeling, it's normal. Don't bottle it up! Talk to family, friends, a counselor, or someone in a support group. Even a quick phone call can brighten the day.

2. Depression and Anxiety: Know the Signs

CKD raises the risk for depression and anxiety. Watch for changes in sleep, appetite, mood, or interest in favorite hobbies. If these signs linger, let your doctor know—treatment and support work wonders.

3. The Healing Power of Social Connection

Family and friends aren't just nice to have; they're part of your "healthcare team." Let them know how to help—errands, check-ins, or just sharing a laugh. Local community centers, clubs, and faith groups offer activities, while online or in-person support groups connect you with others on a similar path.

4. Loneliness and Grief: It's Okay to Mourn

Loss of friends, changes in health, or independence can hurt. Allow yourself to grieve, but don't go it alone. Consider a pet, enjoy time outdoors, or join a group for support.

5. Planning Ahead: The Gift of Clarity

Making your wishes known (with advance directives and a power of attorney) brings peace of mind. Review plans each year, and don't hesitate to ask for help filling out forms—social workers are experts in these conversations.

6. Tackling Healthcare Costs

Medical bills add up. Review insurance yearly, ask about prescription assistance, and keep all bills organized. Social workers can also connect you to affordable transportation, meals, or home care programs.

Resource Tip:

Some drug companies offer help with medication costs—your pharmacist or doctor can point you in the right direction.

7. Safe and Happy at Home

Want to stay independent? Keep walkways clear, install grab bars, use night lights, and consider a medical alert system if needed. Many community agencies offer help with chores or transportation.

Fun Fact:

Grab bars in the bathroom cut fall risk by up to 50%!

8. Hobbies and Joy—Adapt, Don't Quit

Keep doing what you love—whether gardening, cooking, reading, or puzzles. Invite family or friends to join, or explore new activities through local libraries and senior centers.

9. Brain Health: Use It, Don't Lose It

Stay sharp with reading, puzzles, and conversation. Manage health issues (like high blood pressure) and report any memory changes to your doctor. Even a daily crossword can make a difference!

10. Immune Protection: Your Best Defense

CKD makes infection more likely. Get all recommended vaccines, eat well, wash hands often, and treat cuts quickly. Don't ignore fevers or stubborn coughs—call your doctor.

11. Travel and Special Moments: You Can Still Go!

CKD shouldn't stop you from traveling or celebrating. Plan ahead: bring your medication list, pack snacks, and let restaurants know about dietary needs. Enjoy holidays and social events—one off-plan meal won't derail your progress.

12. Nourishing Your Spirit

Spirituality, mindfulness, and gratitude boost resilience. Whether through prayer, meditation, journaling, or a walk in nature, find what soothes your spirit and brings joy to your days.

Conclusion: "The Art of Living Well—Your CKD Journey, Your Way"

CKD may change routines, but it can't take away your ability to live with joy, purpose, and connection. Every step you take—whether with food, medicine, planning, or laughter—builds resilience. Take pride in your journey, reach out for support, and remember: You are never alone. Every day is a new chance to savor life.

1

Breakfast of Champions

LA Egg Toast

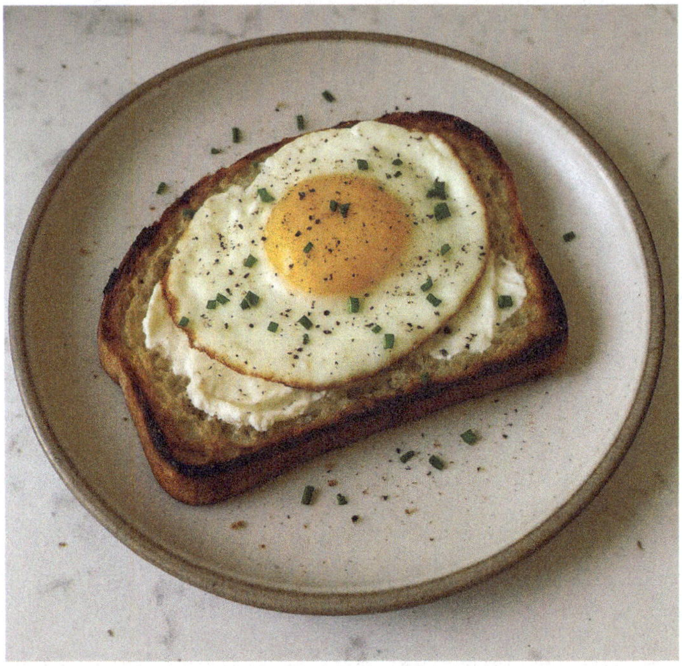

INGREDIENTS

- 1 slice white sourdough bread (low sodium if possible)
- 1 TBL (14g) unsalted butter (for toasting)
- 1 large egg (or pasteurized egg white)
- 2 TBL (30g) cream cheese (low sodium, softened)
- 1 TBL (6g) chives (finely chopped or dried)

DIRECTIONS

1. Toast bread slice in skillet with butter over medium heat until golden on both sides.
2. While bread toasts, cook egg in a nonstick skillet until set (over easy or hard, as preferred).
3. Spread cream cheese over toasted bread.
4. Top with cooked egg.
5. Sprinkle with chives and cracked pepper to taste.

Servings: 1 | Prep Time: 7′ | Cook time: 6′

PROTEIN: MID | PHOSPHORUS: LOW | SODIUM: LOW | POTASSIUM: LOW

CREATIVITY TWIST:
Add fresh dill or swap chives for parsley. Dust with smoked paprika for extra flavor.

Nutritional Info (per serving)
Calories: ~320 kcal | Protein: 14g | Potassium: 175mg | Phosphorus: 120mg | Sodium: 235mg | Fat: 16g | Carbs: 32g | Cholesterol: 215mg | Oxalates: ~8mg

Pacific Cloud Pancakes

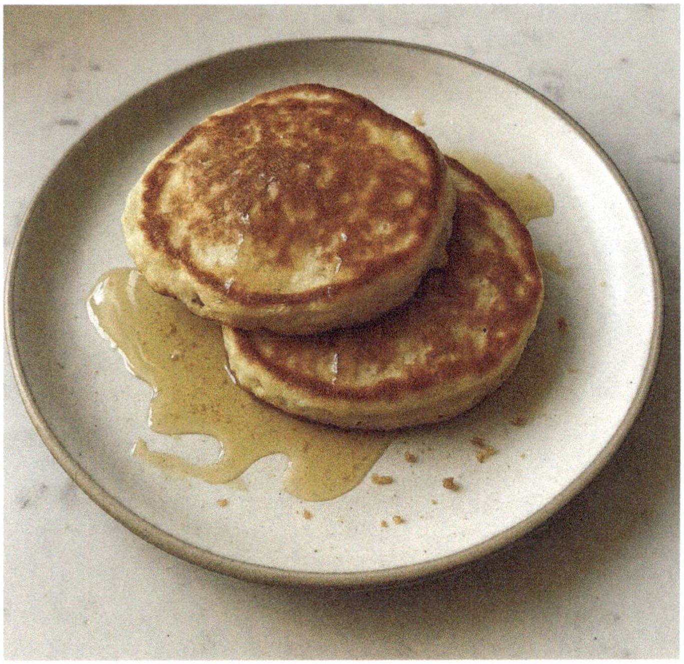

INGREDIENTS

- ½ cup (60g) all-purpose flour
- 1 tsp baking powder
- 1 large egg
- ⅓ cup (80ml) low-fat milk (or oat milk)
- 1 TBL (14g) unsalted butter (for pan)

DIRECTIONS

1. Whisk flour and baking powder in a bowl.
2. In another bowl, beat egg and milk together.
3. Combine wet and dry ingredients, mixing until just smooth.
4. Heat butter in a nonstick pan over medium heat.
5. Spoon batter into pan to form two pancakes.
6. Cook each pancake 2–3 minutes per side until golden brown.
7. Serve warm with a drizzle of honey (optional).

Servings	Prep Time	Cook time
1	10′	10′

PROTEIN	PHOSPHORUS	SODIUM	POTASSIUM
MID	LOW	LOW	LOW

CREATIVITY TWIST:
Top with fresh blueberries or dust with cinnamon. Add a dash of vanilla extract to the batter.

Nutritional Info (per serving)
Calories: ~295 kcal | Protein: 11g | Potassium: 130mg | Phosphorus: 105mg | Sodium: 180mg | Fat: 8g | Carbs: 43g | Cholesterol: 170mg | Oxalates: ~12mg

Sopot Omelette Muffins

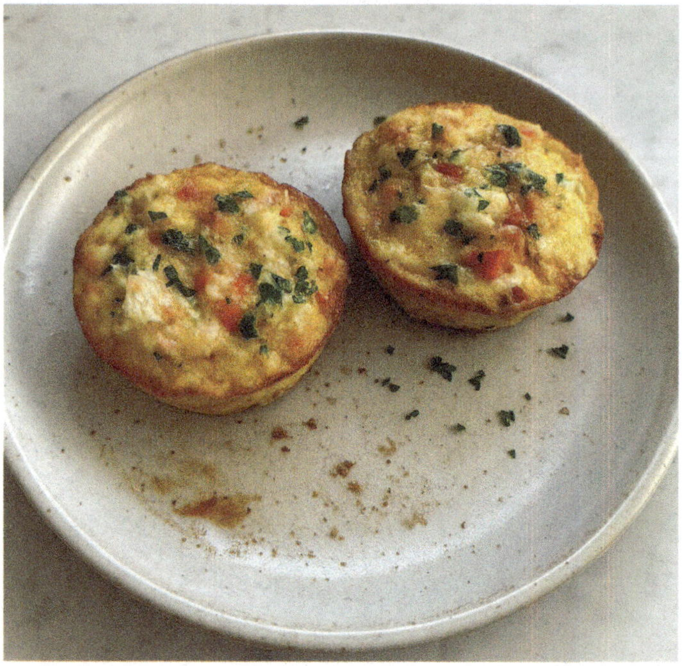

INGREDIENTS

- 2 large eggs
- 2 TBL (30g) cooked crab meat (or cooked white fish, well-drained)
- 2 TBL (30g) ricotta cheese (low sodium)
- 1 TBL (15g) finely diced sweet red bell pepper (peeled)
- 1 TBL (6g) chopped fresh parsley

DIRECTIONS

1. Preheat oven to 350°F (180°C). Grease two muffin cups.
2. Beat eggs in a bowl.
3. Mix in crab meat, ricotta, bell pepper, and parsley.
4. Divide mixture evenly into muffin cups.
5. Bake 10 minutes or until puffed and set.
6. Cool slightly before serving.

Servings	Prep Time	Cook time
2	8'	10'

PROTEIN	PHOSPHORUS	SODIUM	POTASSIUM
MID	LOW	LOW	LOW

CREATIVITY TWIST:
Swap crab for flaked salmon. Use dill and tarragon instead of parsley for French flair.

Nutritional Info (per serving)
Calories: ~160 kcal | Protein: 13g | Potassium: 155mg | Phosphorus: 95mg | Sodium: 170mg | Fat: 9g | Carbs: 2g | Cholesterol: 210mg | Oxalates: ~6mg

Maple Manhattan Cottage Bowl

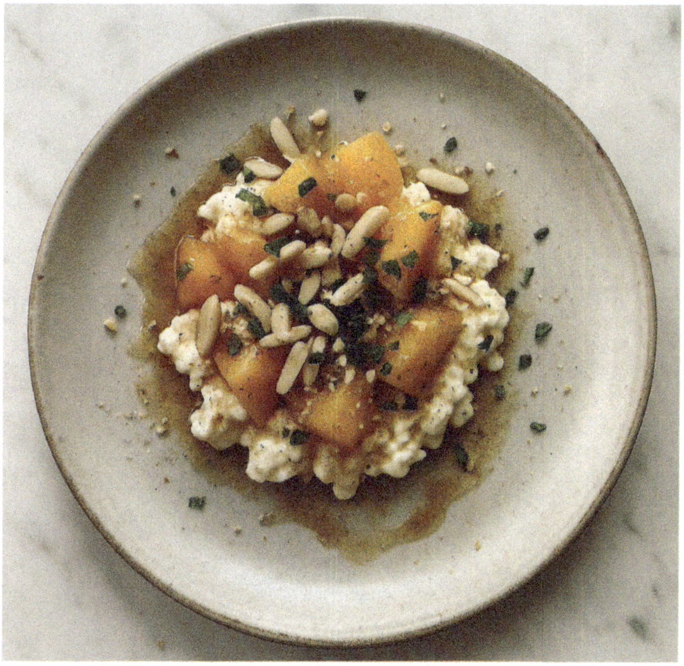

INGREDIENTS

- ½ cup (100g) low-fat cottage cheese (low sodium)
- ½ cup (60g) canned peaches in juice, drained and chopped
- 1 TBL (8g) slivered almonds (raw or lightly toasted)
- 1 tsp maple syrup
- 1 TBL (6g) finely chopped mint

Servings 1 | Prep Time 5' | Cook time 0'

PROTEIN MID | PHOSPHORUS LOW | SODIUM LOW | POTASSIUM LOW

DIRECTIONS

1. In a bowl, layer cottage cheese and peaches.
2. Top with slivered almonds.
3. Drizzle maple syrup over top.
4. Sprinkle chopped mint (and pepper if desired)..

CREATIVITY TWIST:
Swap peaches for pears or pineapple. Add cinnamon or nutmeg for warmth.

Nutritional Info (per serving)
Calories: ~210 kcal | Protein: 13g | Potassium: 190mg | Phosphorus: 110mg | Sodium: 120mg | Fat: 6g | Carbs: 27g | Cholesterol: 10mg | Oxalates: ~14mg

2
Lunch Bunch Favorites

Liberty Garden Chicken Salad

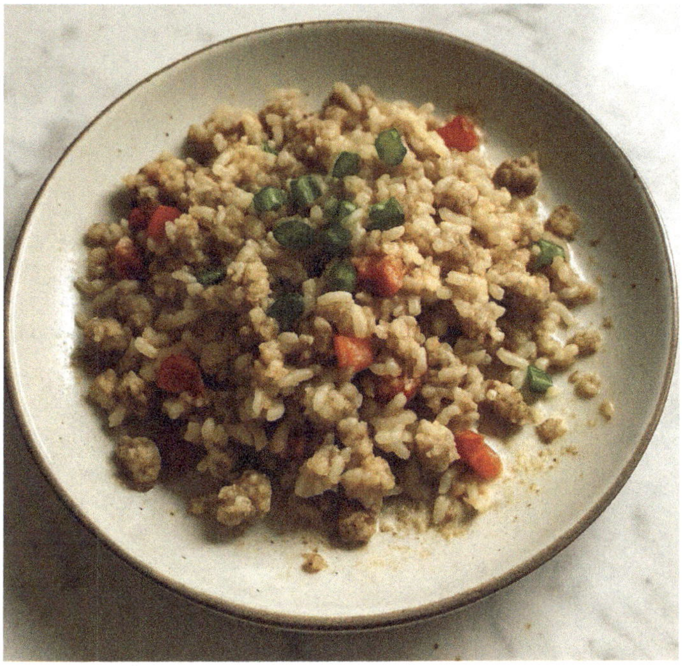

INGREDIENTS

- 1 cup cooked chicken breast, diced (skinless, low sodium) (120g)
- ½ cup seedless red grapes, halved (60g)
- 2 TBL mayonnaise (low sodium)
- 2 TBL chopped celery (peeled if needed)
- 1 TBL chopped fresh dill (or parsley)

DIRECTIONS

1. In a bowl, mix diced chicken, grapes, celery, and dill.
2. Stir in mayonnaise until coated.
3. Serve chilled on a plate or with a slice of white bread.

Servings	Prep Time	Cook time
2	10’	0’

PROTEIN	PHOSPHORUS	SODIUM	POTASSIUM
MID	LOW	LOW	LOW

CREATIVITY TWIST:
Add a squeeze of lemon juice or swap grapes for apple cubes. Try tarragon for a French bistro vibe.

Nutritional Info (per serving)
Calories: ~220 kcal | Protein: 22g | Potassium: 190mg | Phosphorus: 125mg | Sodium: 180mg | Fat: 9g | Carbs: 10g | Cholesterol: 52mg | Oxalates: ~8mg

St. Louis Turkey & Rice Skillet

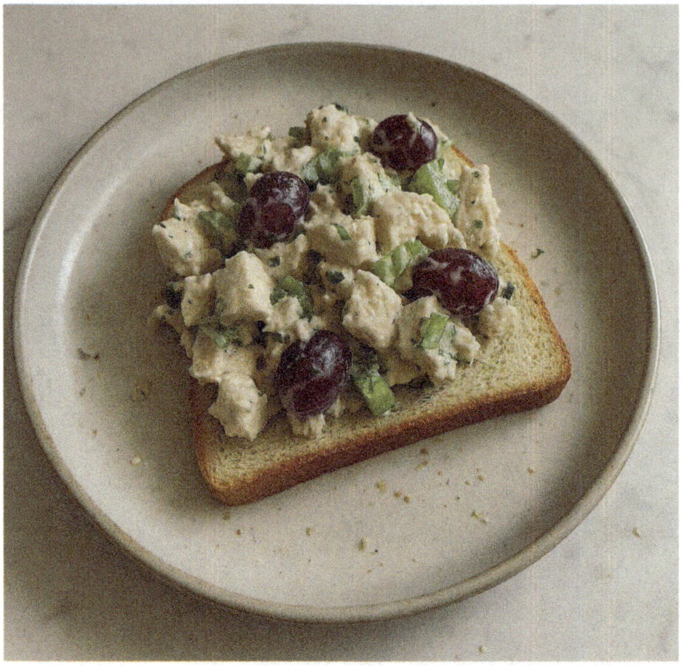

INGREDIENTS

- ⅓ lb ground turkey (lean) (150g)
- 1 cup cooked white rice (185g)
- ¼ cup diced sweet bell pepper
- 2 TBL finely chopped green onions (green tops only)
- 2 TBL olive oil

DIRECTIONS

1. Heat olive oil in a large skillet over medium heat.
2. Add turkey; cook, breaking up, until browned.
3. Add bell pepper and green onion; sauté 2 minutes.
4. Stir in rice and cook until heated through.
5. Season with pepper and serve warm

Servings	Prep Time	Cook time
2	8'	12'

PROTEIN	PHOSPHORUS	SODIUM	POTASSIUM
MID	LOW	LOW	LOW

CREATIVITY TWIST:
Add chopped parsley, a dash of smoked paprika, or finish with a squeeze of lemon for brightness.

Nutritional Info (per serving)
Calories: ~280 kcal | Protein: 22g | Potassium: 185mg | Phosphorus: 130mg | Sodium: 65mg | Fat: 15g | Carbs: 22g | Cholesterol: 63mg | Oxalates: ~7mg

Golden Gate Tuna & Egg Bowlt

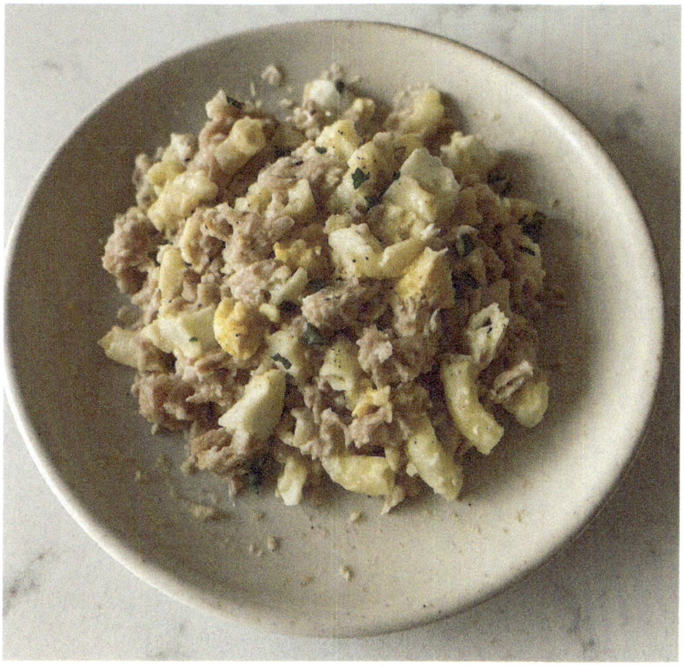

INGREDIENTS

- ½1 can low sodium light tuna in water, drained (3.2 oz / 90g)
- 2 large eggs
- ½ cup cooked macaroni (about 2.3 oz / 66g)
- 1 TBL mayonnaise (low sodium)
- 1 TBL chopped fresh parsley

DIRECTIONS

1. Hard boil eggs (8 min in boiling water), peel and chop.
2. In a bowl, combine tuna, eggs, cooked macaroni, and parsley.
3. Mix with mayonnaise and season with pepper.
4. Serve slightly chilled or at room temperature.

Servings	Prep Time	Cook time
2	6’	8’

PROTEIN	PHOSPHORUS	SODIUM	POTASSIUM
MID	LOW	LOW	LOW

CREATIVITY TWIST:
Try adding a dash of Dijon mustard or swap parsley for fresh dill. Add diced cucumber for extra freshness.

Nutritional Info (per serving)
Calories: ~220 kcal | Protein: 23g | Potassium: 190mg | Phosphorus: 145mg | Sodium: 170mg | Fat: 8g | Carbs: 20g | Cholesterol: 190mg | Oxalates: ~10mg

Charleston Ham & Apple Melt

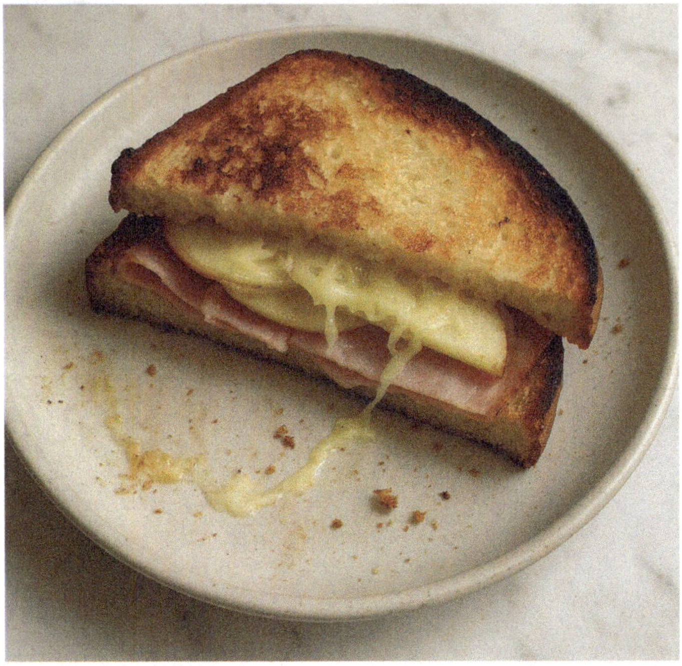

INGREDIENTS

- 1 slice low-sodium ham (1.4 oz / 40g)
- 1 slice white bread (sourdough or sandwich)
- 2 TBL shredded Swiss cheese (low sodium if possible)
- 2 TBL apple slices (peeled, thinly sliced)
- 1 TBL unsalted butter

DIRECTIONS

1. Preheat oven broiler (or use toaster oven).
2. Butter bread and top with ham, apple, and Swiss cheese.
3. Broil until cheese melts (about 3–4 minutes).
4. Cool slightly, slice in half, and serve warm.

Servings: 1 | Prep Time: 5' | Cook time: 8'

PROTEIN: MID | PHOSPHORUS: LOW | SODIUM: LOW | POTASSIUM: LOW

CREATIVITY TWIST:
Swap apple for pear, or add a pinch of nutmeg for a cozy, autumn flavor. Try a sprinkle of fresh thyme for a gourmet touch.

Nutritional Info (per serving)
Calories: ~290 kcal | Protein: 16g | Potassium: 175mg | Phosphorus: 110mg | Sodium: 250mg | Fat: 13g | Carbs: 25g | Cholesterol: 37mg | Oxalates: ~6mg

3
Dinner Time Darling

Savannah Lemon Herb Chicken Medallions

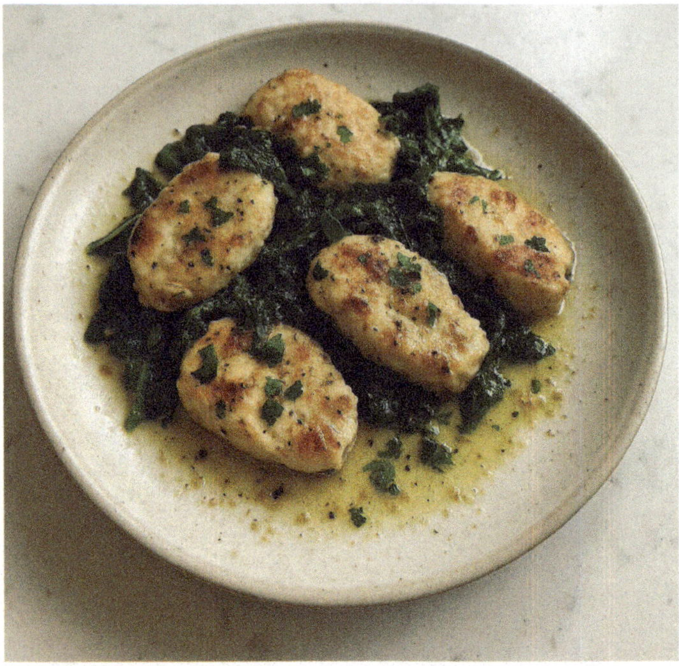

INGREDIENTS

- ⅓8 oz (225 g) chicken breast, thinly sliced
- 1 tbsp olive oil (plus extra for pan)
- 1 small lemon (zest & juice)
- 1.5 oz (40 g) baby spinach (or kale, chopped)
- 2 tbsp chopped fresh parsley

Servings: 2
Prep Time: 8'
Cook time: 15'

DIRECTIONS

1. Pat chicken dry; season with lemon zest, black pepper, and ½ tbsp olive oil.
2. Heat nonstick pan over medium; add remaining oil and chicken. Sear 2–3 mins per side until golden.
3. Add lemon juice and spinach; cook until spinach wilts (~2 mins).
4. Sprinkle with fresh parsley before serving.

PROTEIN: MID
PHOSPHORUS: LOW
SODIUM: LOW
POTASSIUM: LOW

CREATIVITY TWIST:
Swap parsley for fresh dill, or finish with a touch of honey for a sweet-savory note

Nutritional Info (per serving)
Calories: 265 kcal | Protein: 27g | Potassium: 365mg | Phosphorus: 140mg | Sodium: 88mg | Fat: 11g | Carbs: 4g | Cholesterol: 68mg | Oxalates: 16mg

Pacific Bay Salmon Cakes

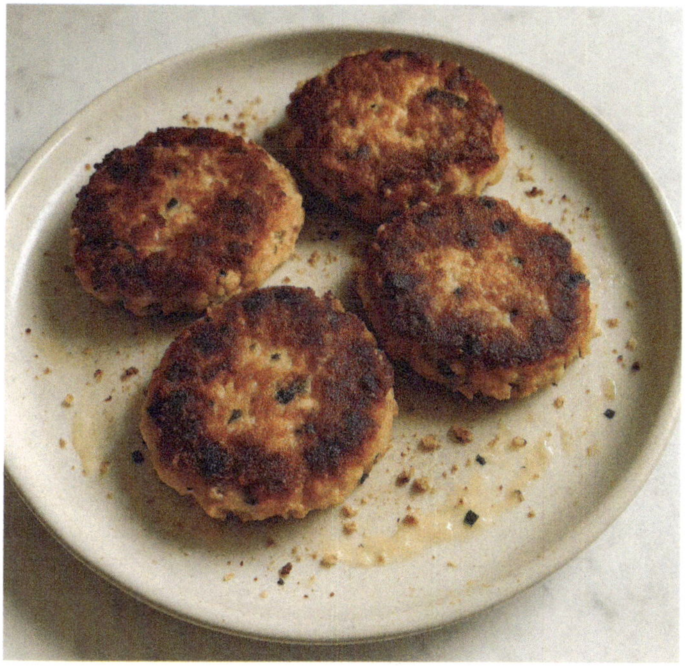

INGREDIENTS

- 6 oz (170 g) canned salmon (drained, bones removed)
- 1 large egg
- 1.5 oz (40 g) panko breadcrumbs (or low sodium cracker crumbs)
- 2 tbsp mayonnaise (low sodium)
- 1 tbsp chopped chives or green onion (white part only)

Servings 2 | Prep Time 6′ | Cook time 8′

PROTEIN MID | PHOSPHORUS LOW | SODIUM LOW | POTASSIUM LOW

DIRECTIONS

1. In a bowl, mix salmon, egg, breadcrumbs, mayo, and chives until just combined.
2. Form into 4 small patties.
3. Heat nonstick skillet with a little olive oil. Cook patties 3–4 mins per side until golden and heated through.

CREATIVITY TWIST:
Serve with a dollop of Greek yogurt and dill, or swap chives for minced tarragon for a French twist.

Nutritional Info (per serving)
Calories: 320 kcal | Protein: 22g | Potassium: 270mg | Phosphorus: 185mg | Sodium: 170mg | Fat: 15g | Carbs: 14g | Cholesterol: 102mg | Oxalates: 12mg

Tuscan Turkey & Zucchini Skillet

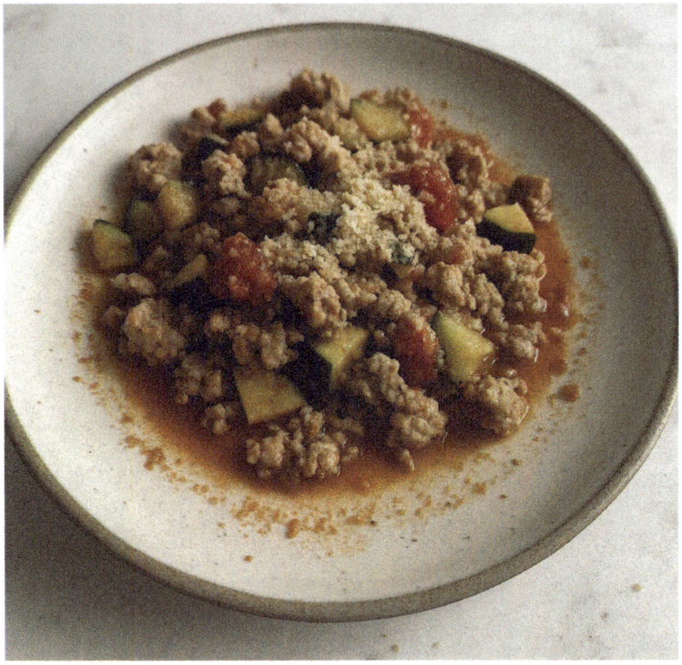

INGREDIENTS

- 8 oz (225 g) ground turkey (lean)
- 1 small zucchini (120 g), diced
- ⅓ cup (80 g) unsalted canned diced tomatoes (drained)
- 2 tbsp grated parmesan (or 2 tsp nutritional yeast for lower phosphorus)
- 1 clove garlic, minced

Servings 2 | Prep Time 7' | Cook time 12'

DIRECTIONS

1. Cook turkey in skillet over medium heat until just browned, breaking up with spoon.
2. Add garlic, zucchini, and tomatoes; sauté until zucchini is soft (~5 mins).
3. Stir in parmesan or nutritional yeast; cook 1 min, then serve.

PROTEIN MID | PHOSPHORUS LOW | SODIUM LOW | POTASSIUM LOW

CREATIVITY TWIST:
Add fresh basil at the end, or a pinch of Italian herbs for extra flavor.

Nutritional Info (per serving)
Calories: 298 kcal | Protein: 24g | Potassium: 352mg | Phosphorus: 158mg | Sodium: 110mg | Fat: 13g | Carbs: 9g | Cholesterol: 83mg | Oxalates: 10mg

Midwest Pork Tenderloin Medallions with Apples

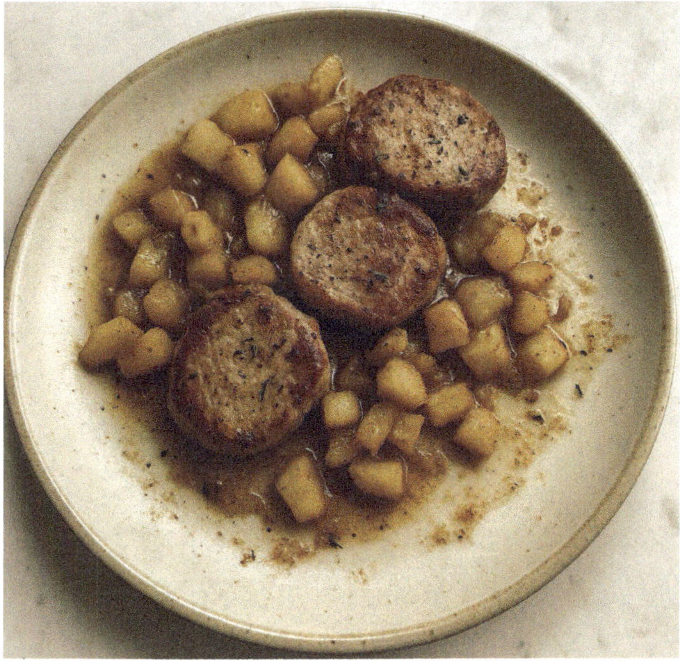

INGREDIENTS

- 8 oz (225 g) pork tenderloin, sliced into 2 cm medallions
- 1 small apple, peeled and diced
- 1 tbsp unsalted butter
- 1 tsp fresh thyme (or ½ tsp dried)
- 1 tbsp apple cider vinegar

DIRECTIONS

1. Season pork with pepper and thyme.
2. Heat butter in skillet on medium-high; sear pork medallions 2–3 mins per side until golden. Remove and keep warm.
3. Add apple to pan; sauté until soft (~2 mins). Stir in vinegar.
4. Return pork to pan; cook 1 min, then serve.

Servings	Prep Time	Cook time
2	8'	11'

PROTEIN	PHOSPHORUS	SODIUM	POTASSIUM
MID	LOW	LOW	LOW

CREATIVITY TWIST:
Try pear instead of apple, or sprinkle with cinnamon for a cozy finish

Nutritional Info (per serving)
Calories: 295 kcal | Protein: 23g | Potassium: 270mg | Phosphorus: 154mg | Sodium: 56mg | Fat: 13g | Carbs: 13g | Cholesterol: 72mg | Oxalates: 8mg

Are you finding this book helpful? I'd love to hear what you think.

If you have just 30 seconds, would you leave a quick review?

It truly makes a huge difference for a small author like me—and it helps other CKD warriors discover this book too.

Here's how you can leave a review for the paperback:

- Option 1: Scan the QR code to go straight to the review page.
- Option 2: Go to your Amazon orders (https://www.amazon.com/orders), find this book, and click "Write a product review."
- Option 3: Search for the book on Amazon, scroll down to the "Customer Reviews" section, and click "Write a Review."

Once you're there, just choose a star rating, jot down a sentence or two about your experience, and click submit!

I personally read every review, and your feedback means the world to me.

Thank you so much for your support.

Scan this with your phone and leave your feedback, I can't wait to read it!

4

Smoothie Smile

New England Berry Cream Dream

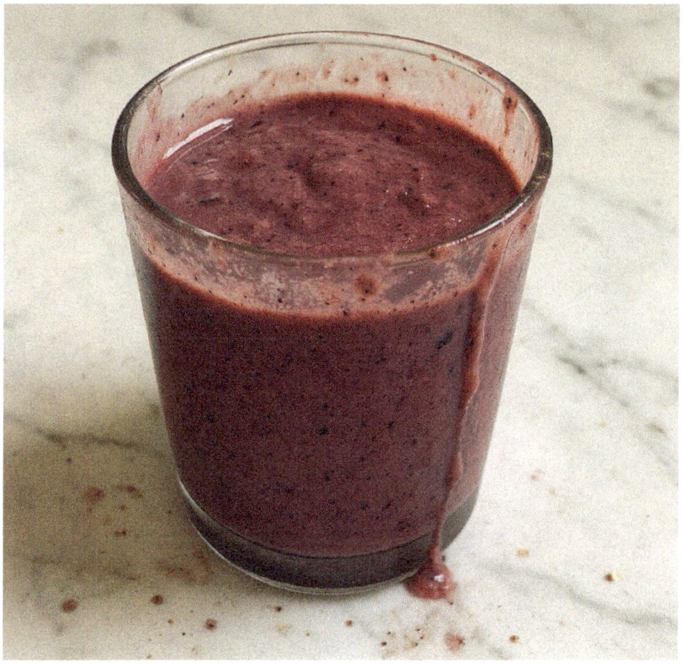

INGREDIENTS

- cup (100 g) frozen blueberries
- ¼ cup (60 g) frozen strawberries
- ½ cup (120 ml) rice milk (unsweetened)
- ¼ cup (60 g) vanilla Greek yogurt (low-fat)
- 1 tsp honey

DIRECTIONS

1. Add all ingredients to a blender.
2. Blend until smooth. Add a splash more rice milk for thinner texture if desired.

Servings	Prep Time	Cook time
2	5'	0'

PROTEIN	PHOSPHORUS	SODIUM	POTASSIUM
LOW	LOW	LOW	LOW

CREATIVITY TWIST:
Swap blueberries for blackberries, or add fresh mint leaves for an herbal note.

Nutritional Info (per serving)
Calories: 145 kcal | Protein: 5g | Potassium: 180mg | Phosphorus: 65mg | Sodium: 44mg | Fat: 1.5g | Carbs: 29g | Cholesterol: 4mg | Oxalates: 14mg

Sunset Peach Lassi

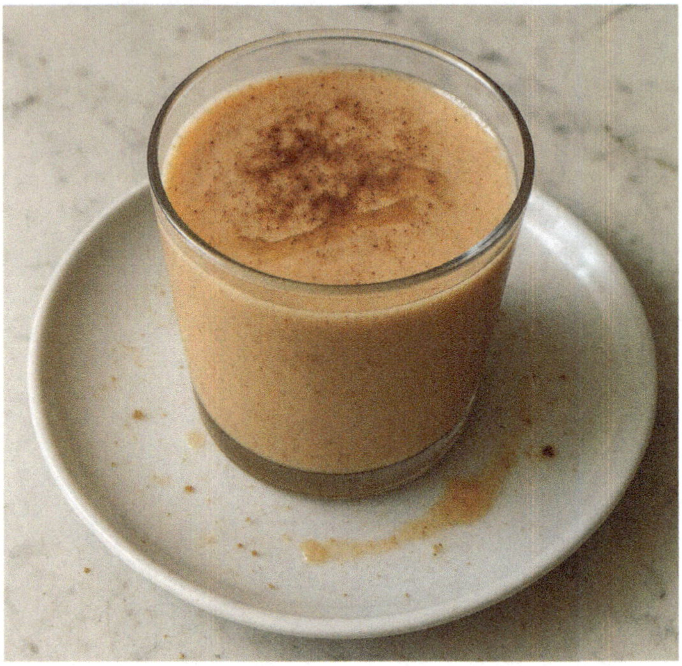

INGREDIENTS

- 1 cup (150 g) frozen peaches
- ½ cup (120 ml) rice milk (unsweetened)
- ¼ cup (60 g) plain Greek yogurt (low-fat)
- ½ tsp ground cinnamon
- 1 tsp honey

DIRECTIONS

1. Place all ingredients in blender.
2. Blend on high until creamy. Add ice for thicker, colder drink.

Servings	Prep Time	Cook time
1	5'	0'

PROTEIN	PHOSPHORUS	SODIUM	POTASSIUM
LOW	LOW	LOW	LOW

CREATIVITY TWIST:
Add a pinch of cardamom, or blend with a couple fresh basil leaves for a refreshing twist.

Nutritional Info (per serving)
Calories: 125 kcal | Protein: 5g | Potassium: 135mg | Phosphorus: 52mg | Sodium: 38mg | Fat: 1.2g | Carbs: 25g | Cholesterol: 3mg | Oxalates: 11mg

Golden Apple Pie Smoothie

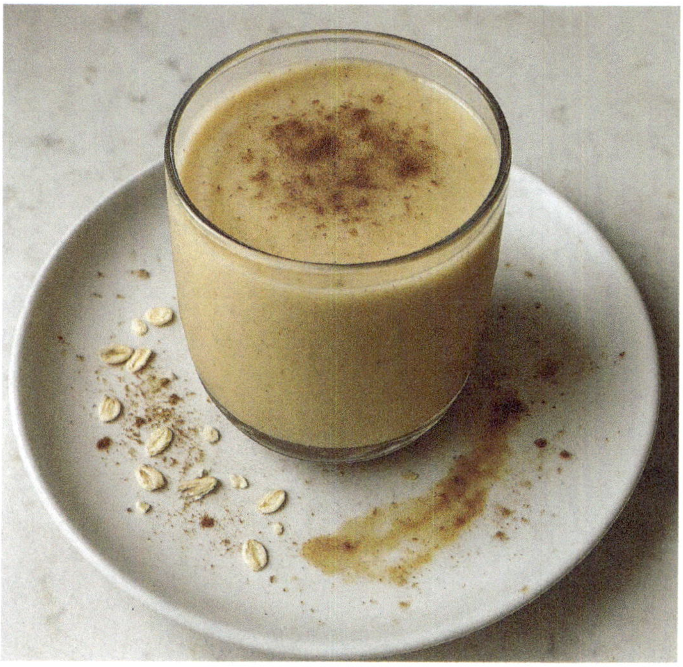

INGREDIENTS

- 8 oz (225 g) pork tenderloin, sliced into 2 cm medallions
- 1 small apple, peeled and diced
- 1 tbsp unsalted butter
- 1 tsp fresh thyme (or ½ tsp dried)
- 1 tbsp apple cider vinegar

DIRECTIONS

1. Season pork with pepper and thyme.
2. Heat butter in skillet on medium-high; sear pork medallions 2–3 mins per side until golden. Remove and keep warm.
3. Add apple to pan; sauté until soft (~2 mins). Stir in vinegar.
4. Return pork to pan; cook 1 min, then serve.

Servings: 1
Prep Time: 5'
Cook time: 0'

PROTEIN: LOW
PHOSPHORUS: LOW
SODIUM: LOW
POTASSIUM: LOW

CREATIVITY TWIST:
Top with a sprinkle of ground nutmeg or a swirl of honey before serving.

Nutritional Info (per serving)
Calories: 128 kcal | Protein: 2.5g | Potassium: 120mg | Phosphorus: 40mg | Sodium: 18mg | Fat: 2g | Carbs: 27g | Cholesterol: 0mg | Oxalates: 7mg

California Creamy Banana-Melon Frappe

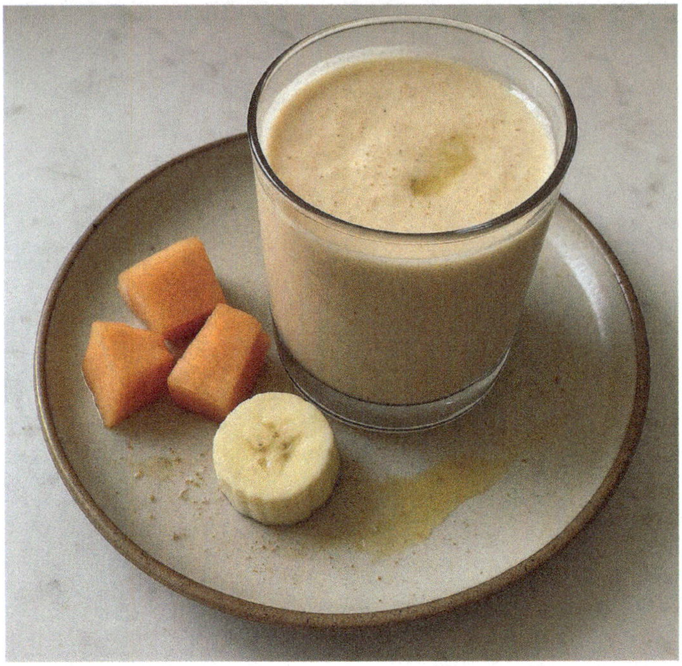

INGREDIENTS

- ½ cup (100 g) fresh or frozen cantaloupe, diced
- ⅓ medium (50 g) ripe banana
- ½ cup (120 ml) rice milk (unsweetened)
- ¼ cup (60 g) vanilla Greek yogurt (low-fat)
- 1 tsp honey

DIRECTIONS

1. Combine all ingredients in blender.
2. Blend until creamy and frothy. Add ice for a colder drink.

Servings 1 | Prep Time 5' | Cook time 0'

PROTEIN LOW | PHOSPHORUS LOW | SODIUM LOW | K POTASSIUM LOW

CREATIVITY TWIST:
Add a dash of vanilla extract, or sprinkle with finely grated ginger for extra zipv

Nutritional Info (per serving)
Calories: 110 kcal | Protein: 4g | Potassium: 150mg | Phosphorus: 42mg | Sodium: 32mg | Fat: 1g | Carbs: 22g | Cholesterol: 2mg | Oxalates: 8mg

5
Sweet Tooth Dessert

Santorini Honey Yogurt Parfait

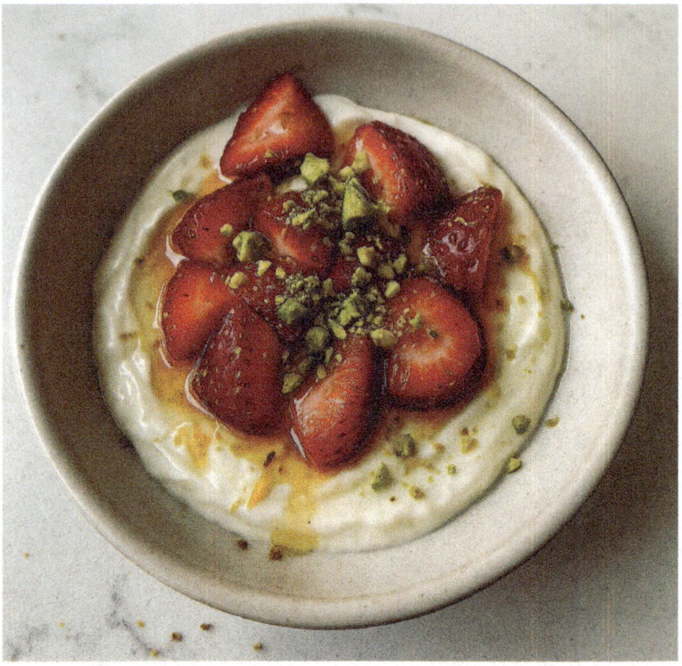

INGREDIENTS

- ¾ cup (150 g) plain Greek yogurt (low-fat)
- ½ cup (60 g) fresh strawberries, sliced
- 2 TBL honey
- 2 TBL (10 g) unsalted shelled pistachios, chopped (optional, for garnish)
- 1 tsp lemon zest

DIRECTIONS

1. Layer yogurt and strawberries in small bowls or glasses.
2. Drizzle with honey and sprinkle lemon zest on top.
3. Garnish with chopped pistachios if desired (omit for lower phosphorus/oxalate).

Servings	Prep Time	Cook time
2	5'	0'

PROTEIN	PHOSPHORUS	SODIUM	POTASSIUM
LOW	LOW	LOW	LOW

CREATIVITY TWIST:
Use blueberries or diced peaches instead of strawberries, or try orange zest for a brighter flavor.

Nutritional Info (per serving)
Calories: 112 kcal | Protein: 6g | Potassium: 112mg | Phosphorus: 47mg | Sodium: 26mg | Fat: 2.8g | Carbs: 17g | Cholesterol: 4mg | Oxalates: 4mg

Valencia Citrus Olive Oil Cakelets

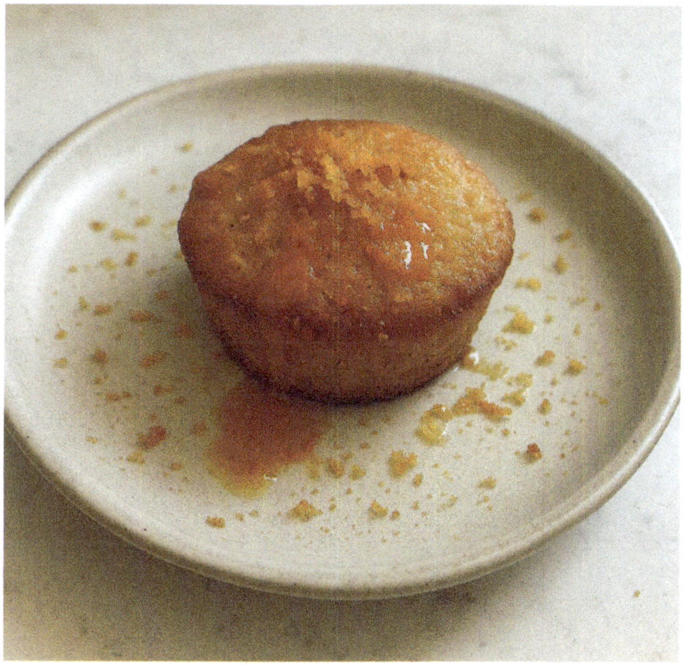

INGREDIENTS

- ¾ cup (90 g) all-purpose flour
- ¼ cup (50 g) granulated sugar
- 1 large egg
- 3 TBL (45 ml) extra virgin olive oil
- 2 TBL orange juice + zest of 1 orange

Servings: 4 mini cakes | Prep Time: 10' | Cook time: 18'

PROTEIN: LOW | PHOSPHORUS: LOW | SODIUM: LOW | POTASSIUM: LOW

DIRECTIONS

1. Preheat oven to 350°F (175°C). Lightly oil mini muffin pan.
2. Whisk egg and sugar in a bowl. Stir in olive oil, orange juice, and zest.
3. Gently fold in flour until just combined.
4. Divide batter among 4 muffin cups. Bake 16–18 mins until golden.
5. Cool and serve with a dusting of zest.

CREATIVITY TWIST:
Top with fruit compote or drizzle honey and fresh mint.

Nutritional Info (per serving)
Calories: 120 kcal | Protein: 2.2g | Potassium: 48mg | Phosphorus: 28mg | Sodium: 13mg | Fat: 5.6g | Carbs: 16g | Cholesterol: 37mg | Oxalates: 2mg

Aegean Rose Rice Pudding

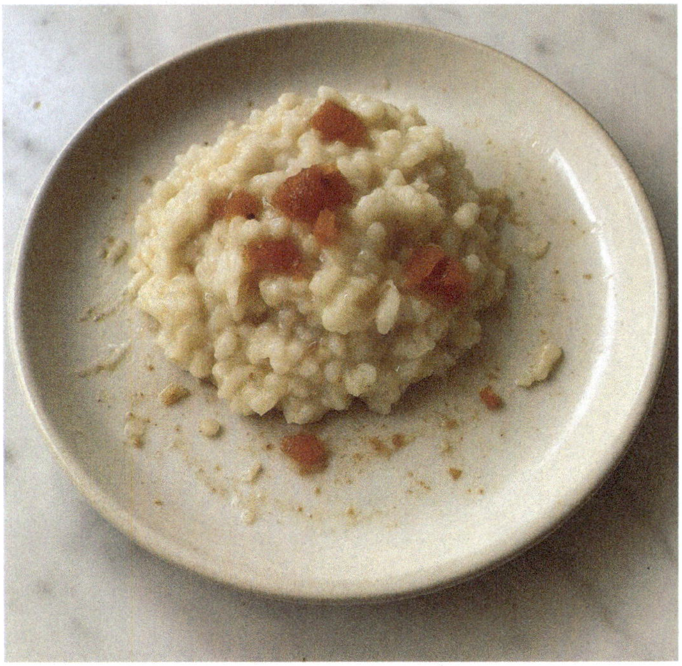

INGREDIENTS

- ¼ cup (50 g) uncooked short-grain rice (e.g., arborio)
- 1 cup (250 ml) rice milk (unsweetened)
- 1 TBL sugar
- 1 tsp rose water
- 1 TBL chopped dried apricots

Servings: 2
Prep Time: 5'
Cook time: 15'

PROTEIN: LOW
PHOSPHORUS: LOW
SODIUM: LOW
POTASSIUM: LOW

DIRECTIONS

1. Combine rice, rice milk, and sugar in saucepan.
2. Simmer gently, stirring often, until rice is tender and pudding thickens (15–18 mins).
3. Stir in rose water and chopped apricots.
4. Cool before serving or serve slightly warm.

CREATIVITY TWIST:
Use orange blossom water instead of rose water, or garnish with chopped pistachios.

Nutritional Info (per serving)
Calories: 113 kcal | Protein: 1.6g | Potassium: 40mg | Phosphorus: 22mg | Sodium: 12mg | Fat: 0.7g | Carbs: 24g | Cholesterol: 0mg | Oxalates: 4mg

Sicilian Lemon Fig Sorbet

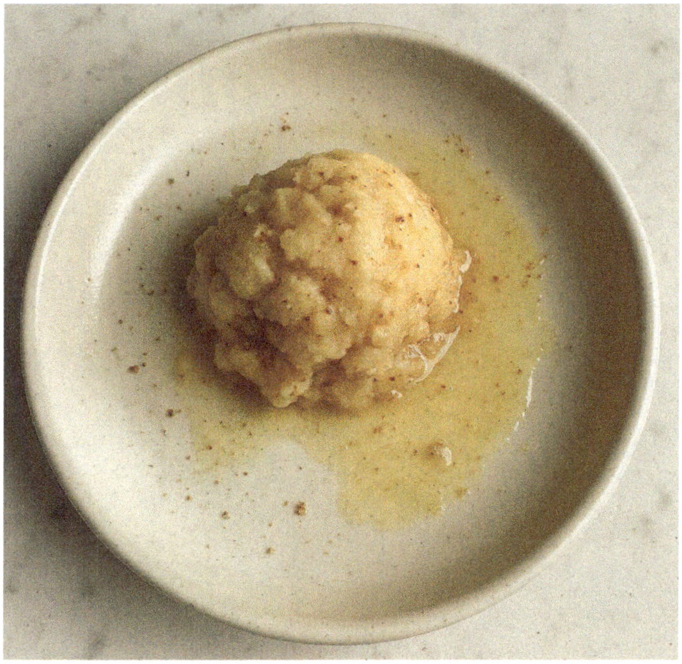

INGREDIENTS

- ¾ cup (120 g) ripe fresh figs, peeled and chopped
- 2 TBL lemon juice
- 2 TBL honey
- ⅓ cup + 1 TBL (100 ml) water
- 1 tsp grated lemon zest

DIRECTIONS

1. Blend figs, lemon juice, honey, water, and lemon zest until smooth.
2. Pour into shallow container and freeze 2–3 hours, stirring every 45 mins for softer texture.
3. Scoop and serve.

Servings	Prep Time	Cook time
2	8' + Freeze	0'

PROTEIN	PHOSPHORUS	SODIUM	POTASSIUM
LOW	LOW	LOW	LOW

CREATIVITY TWIST:
Add fresh basil or mint leaves before blending for a herbal refreshing note.

Nutritional Info (per serving)
Calories: 86 kcal | Protein: 0.7g | Potassium: 82mg | Phosphorus: 17mg | Sodium: 7mg | Fat: 0.2g | Carbs: 21g | Cholesterol: 0mg | Oxalates: 3mg

6

No Grease Airfryer

Nashville Sunrise Egg Bites

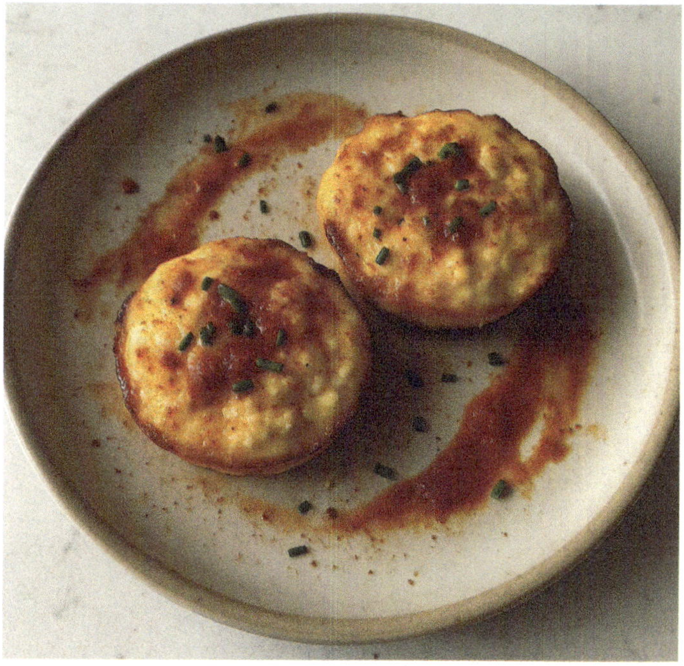

INGREDIENTS

- 4 large eggs
- 2 TBL cottage cheese (low-sodium, low-fat)
- 1 TBL olive oil (for greasing)
- 1/4 tsp smoked paprika
- 1 TBL chopped fresh chives

DIRECTIONS

1. Preheat the air fryer to 325°F (160°C).
2. Lightly grease silicone muffin cups with olive oil.
3. In a bowl, beat eggs, stir in cottage cheese, chives, and paprika.
4. Pour mixture into muffin cups, filling halfway.
5. Air fry for 10 min or until set.
6. Let cool slightly before removing and serving.

Servings 2 | Prep Time 5' | Cook time 10'

PROTEIN MID | PHOSPHORUS LOW | SODIUM LOW | POTASSIUM LOW

CREATIVITY TWIST:
Add a dash of garlic powder or switch to dill for a Scandinavian vibe.

Nutritional Info (per serving)
Calories 220 kcal | Protein 21g | Potassium 260mg | Phosphorus 180mg | Sodium 140mg | Fat 15g | Carb 2g | Chol 360mg | Oxalates: 3mg

Crispy Carolina Chicken Bites

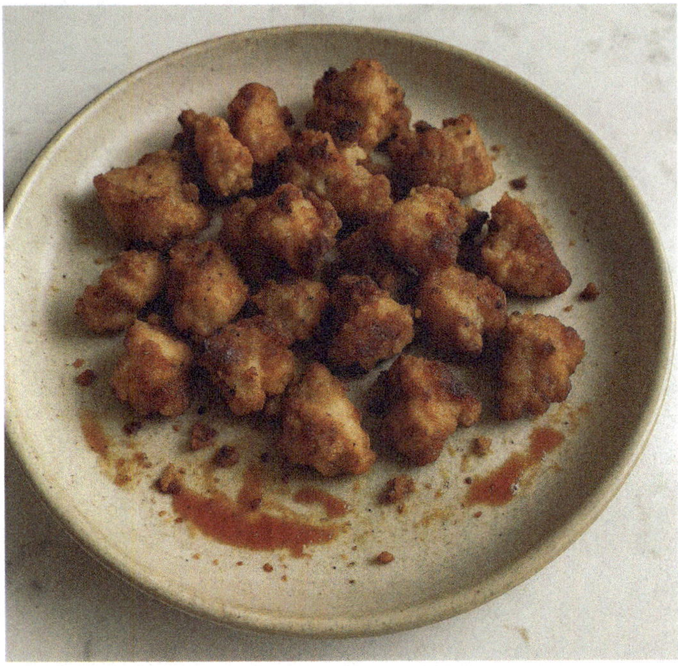

INGREDIENTS

- 200g (7oz) boneless skinless chicken thighs, cut into bite-sized pieces
- 2 TBL all-purpose flour
- 1 TBL olive oil
- 1/4 tsp onion powder
- 1/4 tsp black pepper

Servings 2 | Prep Time 10’ | Cook time 12’

DIRECTIONS

1. Preheat the air fryer to 375°F (190°C).
2. Toss chicken pieces in flour, onion powder, and pepper.
3. Lightly drizzle with olive oil.
4. Place in the air fryer basket, cook for 12 min, shaking halfway through.
5. Serve hot with low-sodium dip or lemon wedge.

PROTEIN MID | PHOSPHORUS LOW | SODIUM LOW | POTASSIUM LOW

CREATIVITY TWIST:
Swap onion powder for za’atar or curry spice for global flair.

Nutritional Info (per serving)
Calories 300 kcal | Protein 23g | Potassium 220mg | Phosphorus 180mg | Sodium 120mg | Fat 17g | Carb 4g | Chol 90mg | Oxalates: 5mg

Florentine Tilapia Crisp

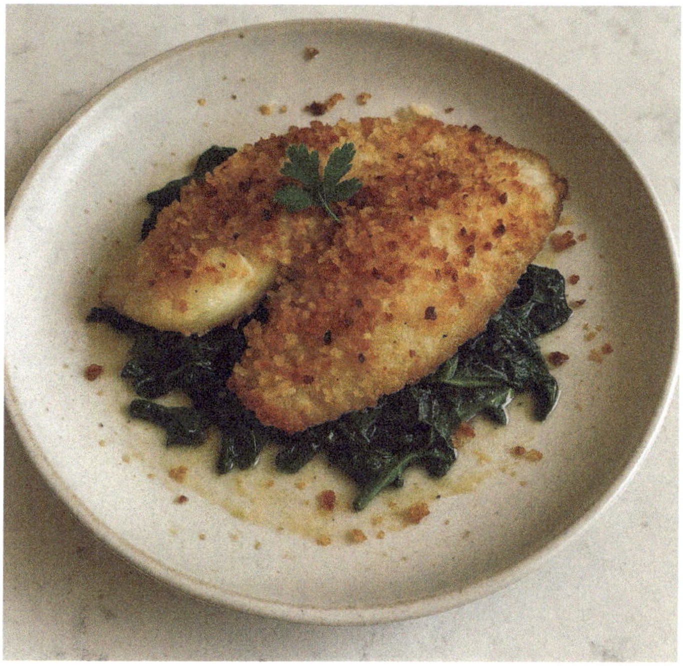

INGREDIENTS

- 2 tilapia fillets (~150g each)
- 2 TBL plain panko breadcrumbs (no salt added)
- 1 TBL lemon juice
- 1 tsp olive oil
- 1/4 tsp garlic powder

DIRECTIONS

1. Preheat the air fryer to 375°F (190°C).
2. Pat fish dry. Brush with lemon juice and oil.
3. Mix panko and garlic powder in bowl, press onto fillets.
4. Air fry for 10 min or until golden and flaky.
5. Serve with parsley or lemon wedge.

Servings	Prep Time	Cook time
2	5'	10'

PROTEIN	PHOSPHORUS	SODIUM	POTASSIUM
MID	LOW	LOW	LOW

CREATIVITY TWIST:
Use crushed cornflakes instead of panko for a crunchier texture.

Nutritional Info (per serving)
Calories 275 kcal | Protein 24g | Potassium 290mg | Phosphorus 160mg | Sodium 95mg | Fat 12g | Carb 3g | Chol 65mg | Oxalates: 3mg

Tuscan Eggplant Rounds

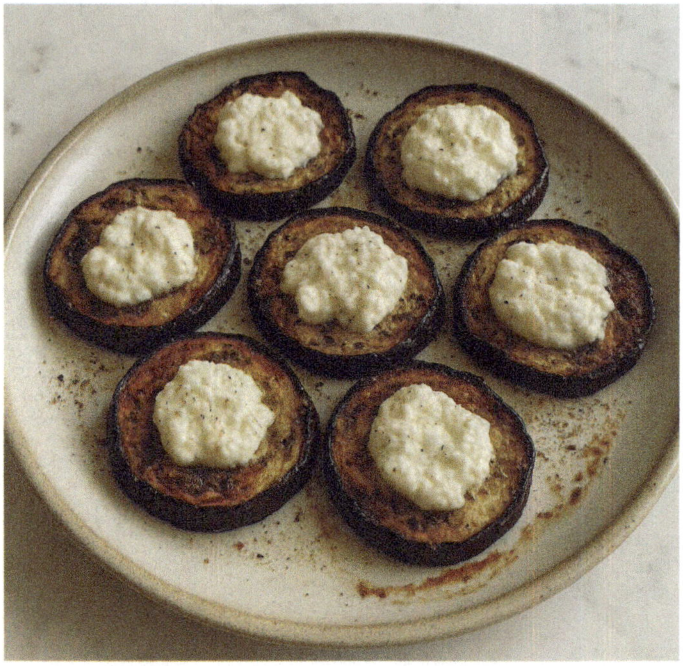

INGREDIENTS

- 1 small eggplant (peeled, sliced 1 cm thick)
- 2 TBL olive oil
- 2 TBL ricotta cheese (low-sodium)
- 1/4 tsp oregano
- 1/4 tsp garlic powder

DIRECTIONS

1. Preheat the air fryer to 350° F (180° C).
2. Brush eggplant slices with olive oil and season with spices.
3. Air fry for 10 min.
4. Top each slice with ricotta, return to the air fryer 5 more min.
5. Serve warm.

Servings	Prep Time	Cook time
2	10'	15'

PROTEIN	PHOSPHORUS	SODIUM	POTASSIUM
LOW	LOW	LOW	LOW

CREATIVITY TWIST:
Add a single fresh basil leaf per round for fragrance and flair

Nutritional Info (per serving)
Calories 200 kcal | Protein 7g | Potassium 280mg | Phosphorus 110mg | Sodium 90mg | Fat 17g | Carb 7g | Chol 15mg | Oxalates: 9mg

Monterey Stuffed Bell Minis

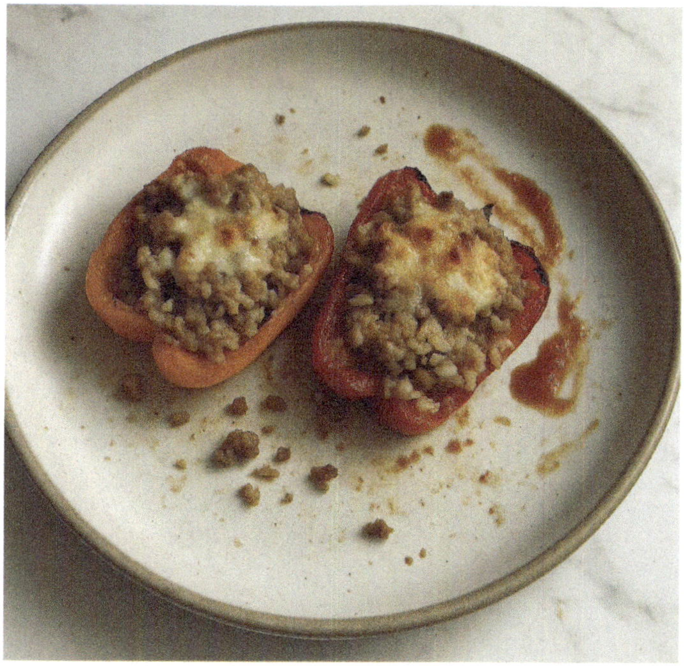

INGREDIENTS

- 2 mini bell peppers (halved, seeds removed)
- 100g lean ground turkey
- 2 TBL cooked white rice
- 1 TBL sour cream (low-fat)
- 1/4 tsp cumin

Servings 2 | Prep Time 10' | Cook time 12'

PROTEIN MID | PHOSPHORUS LOW | SODIUM LOW | POTASSIUM LOW

DIRECTIONS

1. Preheat the air fryer to 370°F (190°C).
2. Cook turkey with cumin in a pan until browned.
3. Mix in the rice and sour cream.
4. Stuff bell pepper halves and place them in the air fryer.
5. Cook for 12 min until peppers are soft.

CREATIVITY TWIST:
Top with fresh parsley or a pinch of paprika before serving

Nutritional Info (per serving)
Calories 290 kcal | Protein 22g | Potassium 390mg | Phosphorus 170mg | Sodium 140mg | Fat 13g | Carb 9g | Chol 55mg | Oxalates: 4mg

Savannah Sweet Potato Wedges

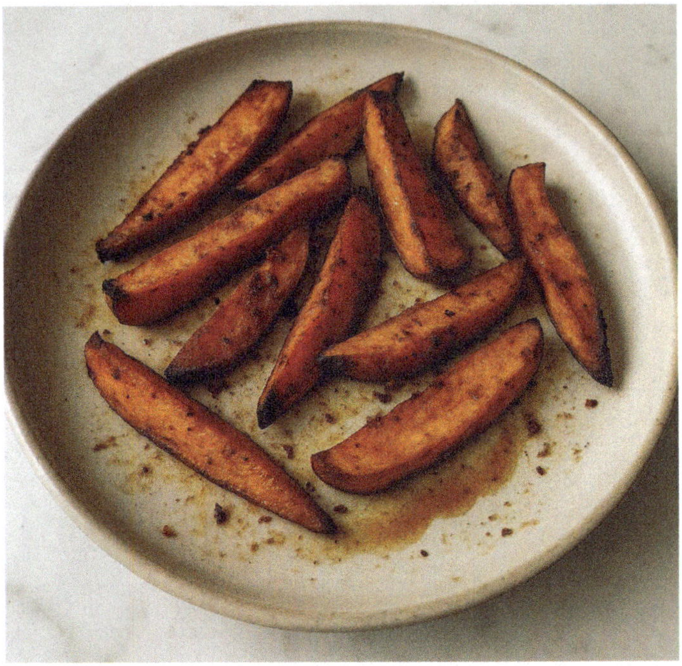

INGREDIENTS

- 1 small sweet potato (peeled, cut into wedges, ~150g)
- 1 TBL olive oil
- 1/4 tsp cinnamon
- 1/4 tsp paprika
- 1 tsp honey

DIRECTIONS

1. Preheat the air fryer to 375°F (190°C).
2. Toss wedges with olive oil, cinnamon, and paprika.
3. Air fry for 15 min, shaking halfway through.
4. Drizzle honey on top before serving.

Servings	Prep Time	Cook time
2	5'	15'

PROTEIN	PHOSPHORUS	SODIUM	POTASSIUM
LOW	LOW	LOW	MID

CREATIVITY TWIST:
Add a tiny pinch of chili flakes for sweet heat contrast.

Nutritional Info (per serving)
Calories 190 kcal | Protein 2g | Potassium 400mg | Phosphorus 60mg | Sodium 30mg | Fat 9g | Carb 28g | Chol 0mg | Oxalates: 15mg

Napoli Mozzarella Zucchini Boats

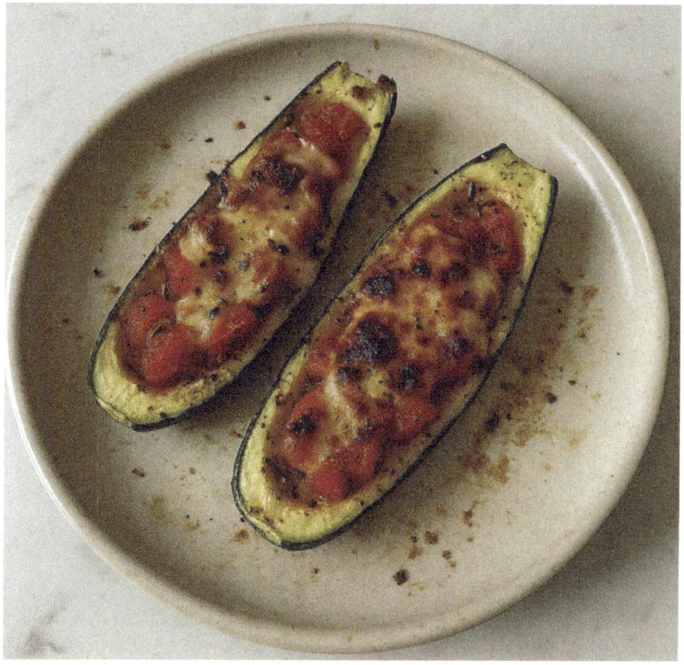

INGREDIENTS

- 1 small zucchini (halved lengthwise, scooped)
- 2 TBL shredded mozzarella (low sodium)
- 1 TBL diced tomato (seeds removed)
- 1 tsp olive oil
- 1/4 tsp Italian seasoning

DIRECTIONS

1. Preheat the air fryer to 370°F (190°C).
2. Brush zucchini halves with oil and sprinkle seasoning on top.
3. Add tomato and cheese into the scooped center.
4. Air fry for 12 min until the cheese is melted and golden.

Servings	Prep Time	Cook time
2	10'	12'

PROTEIN	PHOSPHORUS	SODIUM	POTASSIUM
LOW	LOW	LOW	LOW

CREATIVITY TWIST:
Top with fresh basil or chopped olives for a Mediterranean finish.

Nutritional Info (per serving)
Calories 145 kcal | Protein 6g | Potassium 190mg | Phosphorus 90mg | Sodium 95mg | Fat 11g | Carb 4g | Chol 12mg | Oxalates: 6mg

Brooklyn Apple-Cinnamon Chips

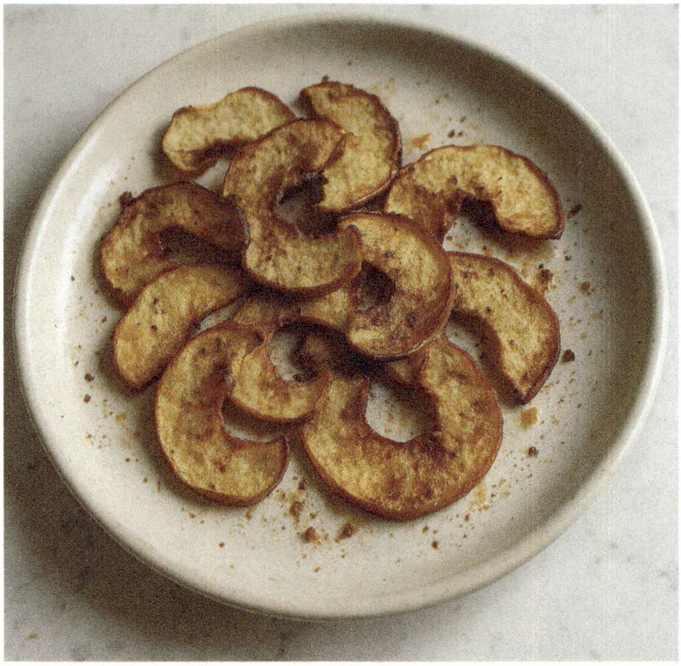

INGREDIENTS

- 1 medium apple (peeled, thinly sliced)
- 1 tsp olive oil
- 1/4 tsp cinnamon
- 1/2 tsp lemon juice
- 1/4 tsp honey

DIRECTIONS

1. Preheat the air fryer to 325°F (160°C).
2. Toss apple slices in oil, cinnamon, and lemon juice.
3. Arrange in a single layer in the basket.
4. Air fry for 12–15 min until crisp.
5. Drizzle with honey before serving.

Servings	Prep Time	Cook time
2	5'	15'

PROTEIN	PHOSPHORUS	SODIUM	POTASSIUM
LOW	LOW	LOW	MID

CREATIVITY TWIST:
Use pear slices and a pinch of ground ginger for variation.

Nutritional Info (per serving)
Calories 95 kcal | Protein 0.3g | Potassium 120mg | Phosphorus 10mg | Sodium 1mg | Fat 3g | Carb 18g | Chol 0mg | Oxalates: 2mg

Barcelona Tuna Patties

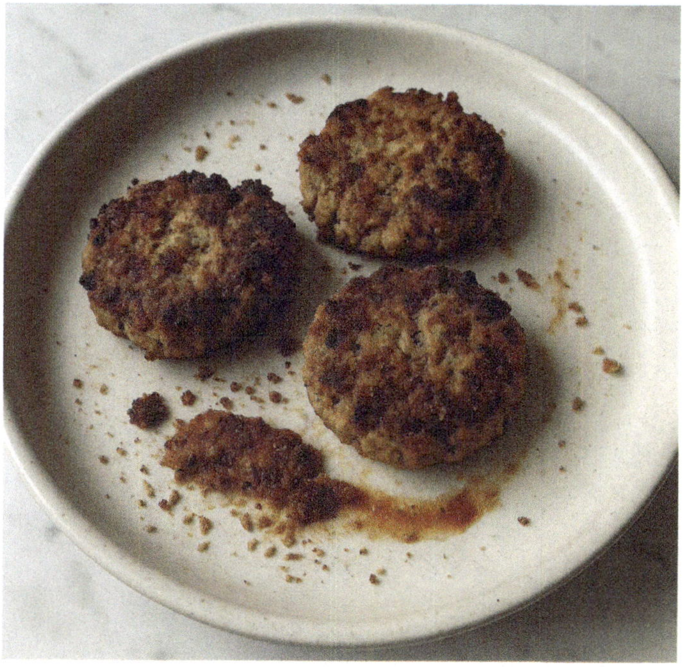

INGREDIENTS

- 1 can low-sodium tuna (drained, ~100g)
- 1 egg
- 2 TBL plain breadcrumbs
- 1 tsp lemon juice
- 1/4 tsp dried dill

Servings: 2
Prep Time: 10'
Cook time: 10'

DIRECTIONS

1. Preheat the air fryer to 370°F (190°C).
2. Mix tuna, egg, breadcrumbs, lemon juice, and dill.
3. Form into 4 small patties.
4. Air fry for 10 min, flipping halfway through.

PROTEIN: MID
PHOSPHORUS: LOW
SODIUM: LOW
POTASSIUM: LOW

CREATIVITY TWIST:
Add a pinch of smoked paprika or serve with cucumber yogurt dip.

Nutritional Info (per serving)
Calories 260 kcal | Protein 22g | Potassium 190mg | Phosphorus 170mg | Sodium 140mg | Fat 12g | Carb 6g | Chol 95mg | Oxalates: 3mg

Parisian Chicken & Apple Skewers

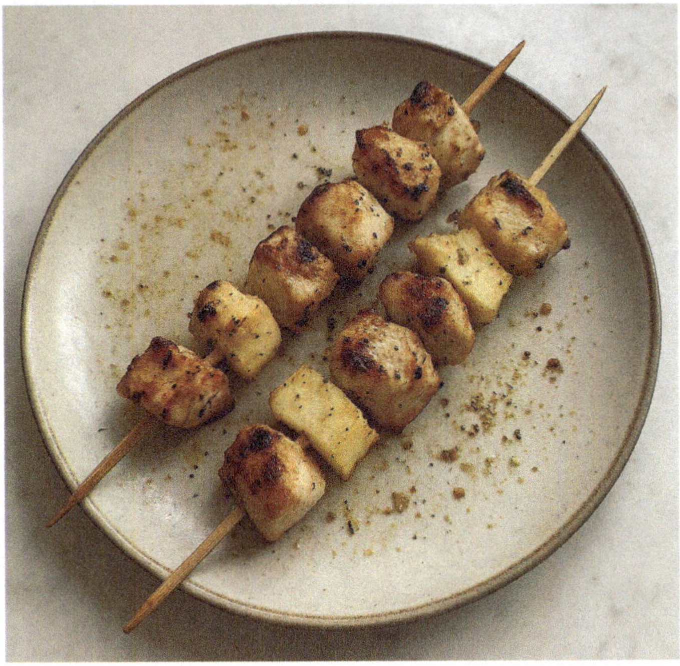

INGREDIENTS

- 200g chicken breast, cubed
- 1 small apple, diced
- 1 TBL olive oil
- 1/4 tsp thyme
- 1/4 tsp black pepper

DIRECTIONS

1. Preheat the air fryer to 375°F (190°C).
2. Thread alternating chicken and apple onto skewers.
3. Brush with oil and sprinkle thyme and pepper on top.
4. Air fry 10 min, turning once.

Servings	Prep Time	Cook time
2	10’	10’

PROTEIN	PHOSPHORUS	SODIUM	POTASSIUM
MID	LOW	LOW	MID

CREATIVITY TWIST:
Add a dash of cinnamon on the apples for sweet-savory contrast.

Nutritional Info (per serving)
Calories 310 kcal | Protein 24g | Potassium 410mg | Phosphorus 180mg | Sodium 120mg | Fat 14g | Carb 10g | Chol 75mg | Oxalates: 4mg

Texas Toasted Tofu Bites

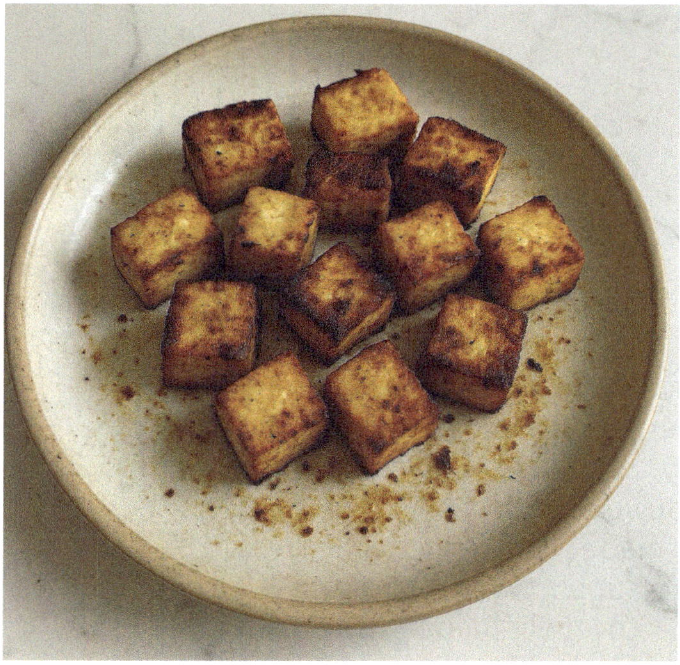

INGREDIENTS

- 200g firm tofu, pressed and cubed
- 1 TBL olive oil
- 1/4 tsp turmeric
- 1/4 tsp garlic powder
- 1 tsp apple cider vinegar

Servings: 2 | Prep Time: 5' | Cook time: 12'

PROTEIN: MID | PHOSPHORUS: LOW | SODIUM: LOW | POTASSIUM: LOW

DIRECTIONS

1. Preheat the air fryer to 370°F (190°C).
2. Toss tofu in a bowl with oil, vinegar, turmeric, and garlic powder.
3. Place in the air fryer basket in a single layer.
4. Air fry 12 min, shaking halfway.

CREATIVITY TWIST:
Add crushed rosemary or lemon zest for a bright herbal finish.

Nutritional Info (per serving)
Calories 280 kcal | Protein 22g | Potassium 260mg | Phosphorus 180mg | Sodium 80mg | Fat 18g | Carb 3g | Chol 0mg | Oxalates: 18mg

Conclusion: What You've Learned and What's Next

Dear Friend,

You've come so far on this journey already. In these pages, you've learned how your kidneys work and what stage 3 CKD means. You've discovered simple, tasty recipes made with everyday ingredients that support your kidney health without overwhelming you. You've gained tools to shop smarter, read labels with confidence, and build daily habits that nurture your whole self—body, mind, and heart.

I know this path isn't always easy. It can feel scary or lonely at times. But please remember, you're not alone. Every step you take, no matter how small, is a powerful act of love toward yourself and those who care about you. You are stronger than you know, and you deserve kindness, patience, and hope every day.

This book is all you need to understand what you need. It's—the place to start when you feel lost or overwhelmed. If you're ready for more, I'm working on a much more comprehensive guide, with over 100+ recipes, 60-day meal plans, expanded nutrition tips, and deeper guidance for caregivers and seniors alike. If you want to be the first to know when it's ready, be sure to sign up for updates by claiming your gift.

AWESOME UPDATE: It just got published!

To see it go to the next page for the QR code.

or use this link:

https://amzn.to/4lrPYoV

I want to invite you to keep walking this path with us—because community makes all the difference. Join our Facebook group, Kidney Disease Warriors: Stage 3 & 4 CKD Diet, Recipes and Community. There, you'll find people who truly understand what you're facing, who share their stories, struggles, and victories, and who are ready to welcome you with open arms. I can't wait to see you there, hear your story, and support you as you continue to live well with CKD.

From my heart to yours, thank you for letting me be part of your journey. We're just getting started.

With all my love,

Marianne Greene <3

Did you find this book helpful? I'd love to hear what you think.

If you have just 30 seconds, would you leave a quick review?

It truly makes a huge difference for a small author like me—and it helps other CKD warriors discover this book too.

Here's how you can leave a review for the paperback:

- Option 1: Scan the QR code to go straight to the review page.
- Option 2: Go to your Amazon orders (https://www.amazon.com/orders), find this book, and click "Write a product review."
- Option 3: Search for the book on Amazon, scroll down to the "Customer Reviews" section, and click "Write a Review."

Once you're there, just choose a star rating, jot down a sentence or two about your experience, and click submit!

I personally read every review, and your feedback means the world to me.

Scan this with your phone and leave your feedback, I can't wait to read it!

Join Our Private Facebook Group!

Living with CKD can feel isolating and overwhelming, especially when it comes to diet and lifestyle changes. In this group, you're not alone. You'll gain support from a community that truly understands what you're facing, get answers to your questions, and feel empowered with encouragement and resources tailored to your needs. Just search

"Kidney Disease Warriors: Stage 3 & 4 CKD Diet, Recipes and Community"

The group is on Facebook—we can't wait to welcome you.

Or Scan this and request to join our group <3

If you haven't Already claimed it, here is your BONUS: Free Kidney-Safe Power Tools

Worried about dining out with Stage 3 Kidney Disease? We've got you covered. Grab your FREE Kidney-Safe Power Tools featuring:

- A game-changing Dining Out Cheat Sheet with smart swaps to order anywhere, red-flag items to avoid, and simple questions to ask your server.
- A CKD do-it-yourself Weekly Meal Planner to stay on track
- A Kidney-Friendly Grocery List for Smart Shopping
- Take control beyond your kitchen by starting with your bonus gift.

Click here to get your bonuses and our next book for FREE:

https://greenhopex.com/dining-out-s3kd

or Scan this QR code to Claim your free gifts:

Simple tools. Big impact. Better living starts in your pantry.

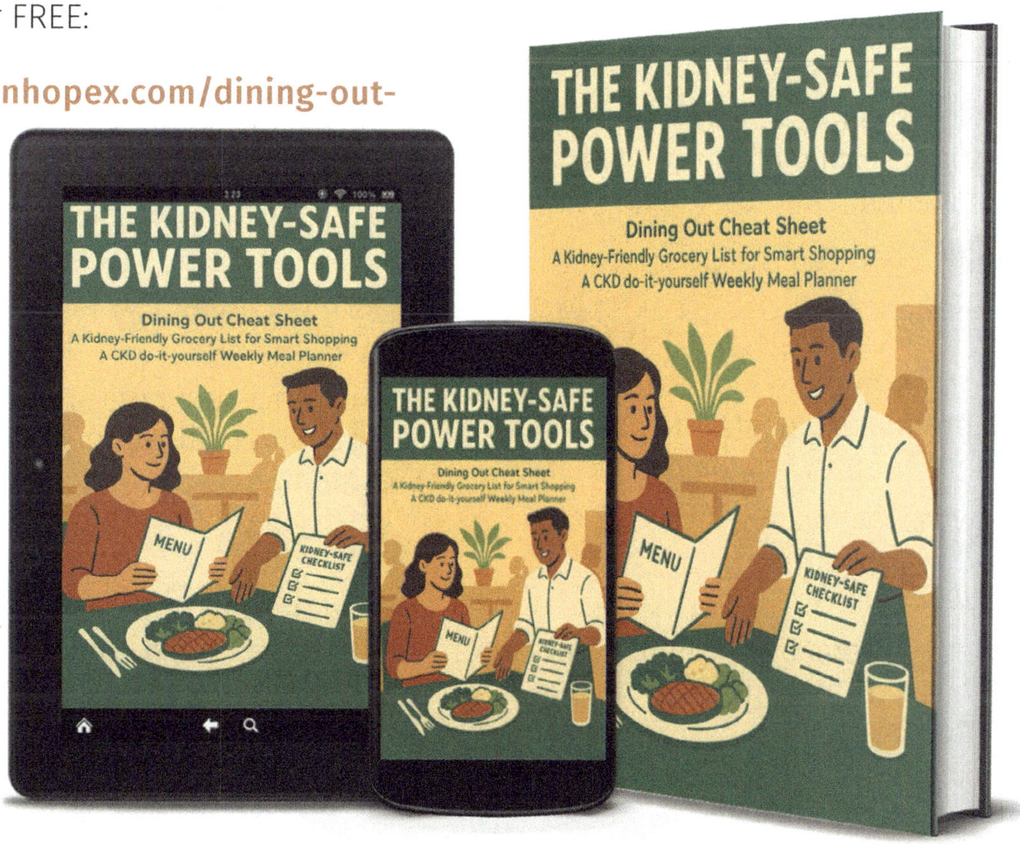

Resources

MEDICAL EDUCATION

National Kidney Foundation (NKF)

Trusted nonprofit offering clear info on CKD stages, tests, treatments, and patient mentoring programs.

www.kidney.org

American Kidney Fund (AKF)

Provides kidney disease education, stage-by-stage guides, and financial aid info for patients.

www.kidneyfund.org

National Institute of Diabetes and Digestive and Kidney Diseases (NIDDK)

Government site with plain-language explanations of CKD causes, management, and diet tips.

niddk.nih.gov

Mayo Clinic – Chronic Kidney Disease

Comprehensive overview of CKD symptoms, diagnosis, and treatment in patient-friendly language.

www.mayoclinic.org

Kidney School

Free, interactive online education modules to learn how to manage CKD day-to-day.

kidneyschool.org

MedlinePlus – Chronic Kidney Disease

NIH consumer health site offering easy summaries, videos, and links to kidney resources.

medlineplus.gov

RENAL DIET AND MEAL PLANNING

American Kidney Fund – Kidney Kitchen

Kidney-friendly recipes, meal plans, and nutrition guides tailored for CKD diets.

kitchen.kidneyfund.org

DaVita Kidney Care – Diet & Nutrition

Hundreds of renal diet recipes, meal planning tools, and nutrition education.

davita.com/diet-nutrition

National Kidney Foundation – Nutrition Label Reading

Guidance on interpreting food labels for sodium, phosphorus, and potassium content.

www.kidney.org

Academy of Nutrition and Dietetics – Find a Renal Dietitian

Directory to locate registered dietitians specializing in kidney disease.

eatright.org/find-an-expert

Kidney Community Kitchen (Canada)

Kidney-friendly recipes and meal planning tools (metric units, international use).

kidneycommunitykitchen.ca

ONLINE SUPPORT AND COMMUNITY

NKF Kidney Community Forums (HealthUnlocked)

Active online support forums connecting CKD patients, caregivers, and experts.

healthunlocked.com/nationalkidneyfoundation

American Association of Kidney Patients (AAKP) Support Groups

Directory of in-person and virtual support groups for kidney patients and caregivers.

aakp.org/support-groups

Renal Support Network (RSN)

Patient-run nonprofit with monthly virtual support groups, podcasts, and webinars.

rsnhope.org

I Hate Dialysis Forums

Peer-to-peer online message boards for CKD patients and caregivers at all stages.

ihatedialysis.com

Facebook Support Groups

Numerous private Facebook groups offer peer support for CKD patients and families.

Search "Chronic Kidney Disease Support" on Facebook

NKF Cares Helpline

Free kidney health phone support and resource referral at 1-855-653-2273.

FINANCIAL AID AND MEDICATION HELP

American Kidney Fund Financial Assistance

Need-based grants for insurance, treatment, and related expenses for kidney patients.

kidneyfund.org/get-assistance

Medicare and SHIP

Federal and state programs helping cover CKD treatment and medication costs; call 1-800-MEDICARE or contact your local State Health Insurance Assistance Program.

Patient Access Network (PAN) Foundation

Grants for copays and treatment expenses for eligible kidney-related conditions.

panfoundation.org

HealthWell Foundation

Financial aid for medication copays and premiums for certain chronic illnesses including kidney disease.

healthwellfoundation.org

NeedyMeds

Database of prescription assistance programs to help patients afford medications.

needymeds.org

Medicine Assistance Tool (MAT)

Search engine for manufacturer prescription assistance programs by drug name.

medicineassistancetool.org

American Kidney Fund Prescription Discount Card

Free discount card to save on medications without income restrictions.

kidneyfund.org

TOOLS AND TRACKERS

DaVita Diet Helper

Interactive online meal planner that customizes renal diet meal plans and tracks nutrients.

davita.com/diet-helper

Mizu App

Mobile app for CKD patients to track symptoms, diet, and medications with reminders.

Available on iOS and Android app stores (search "Mizu CKD")

CareClinic Symptom Tracker

Mobile app for logging CKD symptoms, medications, and lifestyle habits.

careclinic.io

MediSafe

User-friendly medication reminder app with notifications and logs for patients and caregivers.

Available on iOS and Android app stores

PhosFilter App

iOS app that scans grocery barcodes to detect phosphate additives in foods.

Search "PhosFilter" in Apple App Store

Blood Pressure Monitors with App Sync

Recommended home BP monitors like Omron with apps to track and share blood pressure readings.

Printable CKD Journals

Free downloadable symptom and medication tracking sheets available on NKF and AKF websites.

Made in the USA
Monee, IL
18 October 2026

66036203R00044